FLOWER
ESSENCES

*Reordering Our
Understanding and
Approach To
Illness and Health*

Machaelle Small Wright

FLOWER ESSENCES

Reordering Our
Understanding and
Approach To
Illness and Health

PERELANDRA, LTD.
CENTER FOR NATURE RESEARCH
JEFFERSONTON ✿ VIRGINIA
1988

This book is manufactured in the United States of America.

Designed by Machaelle Small Wright and James F. Brisson.

Cover design by James F. Brisson, Williamsville, VT 05362.

Cover photo by Clarence N. Wright.

Edited by the Window, David, John and Machaelle Wright.

Copy-edited by Beverly Beane, Dublin, NH 03444.

Suggestions by Jane Flemer, Marilyn Holbeck, DC and Susan Kasper.

Legwork, paste-up, computer tech lifesaver, support and meals
by Clarence N. Wright.

Formatting, typesetting and computer wizardry by Machaelle Small Wright.

This book was formatted, laid out and produced using the Xerox Ventura Publisher software along with the Kyocera F-1010 laser printer.

Published by Perelandra, Ltd., P.O. Box 3603, Warrenton, VA 20188.

Printed on recycled paper.

Library of Congress Card Catalog Number: 88-090610

Wright, Machaelle Small

*Flower Essences: Reordering Our Understanding
and Approach to Illness and Health*

ISBN 0-9617713-3-X

897

Table of Contents

To
Brother Butch,
Windows and Nature,
the Cottage-level team,
and the Perelandra-level team.
Ain't it great when all
the pieces come
together.

FLOWER ESSENCES

*Reordering Our
Understanding and
Approach To
Illness and Health*

1

What Are
These Things Called
Flower Essences?

IN 1978 A CHIROPRACTOR recommended to me that I use something called "flower essences." I had absolutely no idea what they were or what they did. He gave me a quick thumbnail description plus an address for the Bach Flower Essences. I still didn't have much of an idea of what these things were, but something rang right inside. So I ordered a set of the Bach Flower Essences from England and got on with the chore of figuring out how to use them, why, and when.

Since then, I have used, studied, and experimented with many essences, and even developed my own flower essences. In the process I have grown to respect them beyond words for their role in health and balance. I've felt what they can do. I've watched what look to be miracles being pulled off in routine ways with the essences. I've had the honor of using essences to help others through illness or other difficult times. And since incorporating them in my life, I've been in a continuous, personal-awareness education program that mirrored back to me who I am, how I react and respond to life, and where my strengths and weaknesses lie.

Needless to say at this point, I am enthusiastic about flower essences. Now I find myself saying to others, "You should be using flower essences." They look at me funny and say, "What are they?" And then I give them the same kind of dumb thumbnail sketch I was given in 1978. Sometimes it clicks with them, sometimes it doesn't. When it doesn't, I have this overwhelming urge to grab them by the neck, shake them silly, and shout, "Don't you understand that these things could be one of the most important things you'll ever incorporate in your life!?" Well, instead of running around and accosting everyone, I've decided to use a different approach. I thought, What if I took the time to explain all that I know and have experienced about the flower essences, including what they are, how to use them, and when to use them. What if I went beyond that thumbnail sketch and gave people real information. Surely this would do the trick.

Hence, this book. Whenever appropriate, I will be including information and insight from the higher intelligences who are associated with the essences and health. I feel that although modern flower essences have been around since the mid-1930s and have been used by professionals and laymen alike with terrific results, we really have only begun to scratch the surface as to what the essences are and how they may be used. I look to these higher intelligences to move me along in my understanding and knowledge — and it is in this spirit (pardon the pun) that I offer their input throughout this book.

One other thing. I have written about flower essences both in the *Perelandra Garden Workbook* and in the *Perelandra Rose and*

Garden Essences Guide. For the sake of clarity and convenience to you, I am including that information here. For those of you who have read the *Workbook* and/or the *Guide*, you may think you are having a déjà-vu experience every once in a while as you read along. Don't get excited. It's probably just one of the sections you've already read.

Now, with all that said, let me alleviate your curiosity and give you the typical introductory thumbnail flower essences sketch. To set this up, you have to ask, "What are flower essences?" Then I say something like, "Flower essences are liquid, pattern-infused solutions made from individual plant flowers, each containing a specific imprint that responds in a balancing, repairing, and re-building manner to imbalances in humans on their physical, emotional, mental, and spiritual or universal levels."

Why we who love the essences think that the above is an easily comprehensible answer is beyond me. But this is the kind of answer one gets hit with. As a matter of fact, this is the opening sentence in the *Perelandra Rose and Garden Essences Guide*. The problem is, it's accurate — just intellectual and a little out of reach. So let me try again.

I have learned from the nature intelligences I work with that specific healing and balancing patterns that are vital to humans have been incorporated in the makeup of plant life. These patterns are usually found in the flower petals of the plant. When the petals are placed in water and allowed to sit in the sun for a period of about three hours, that specific healing and balancing pattern is released into the water in a highly condensed form. The water is now what can be called a "tincture." The tincture is diluted, preserved, usually in brandy, and is then ready to be taken orally a few drops at a time whenever needed.

How does this link in with the human body? We humans borrow from the three kingdoms in nature what is needed for an appropriate physical form. It stands to reason. Everything that is of form on Earth is derived from nature. We draw from the animal kingdom for our physical form and from the mineral kingdom for the building and stabilizing process in our cells. And for our central nervous system, we draw from the plant kingdom. Because of their close relationship, the central nervous system responds easily and favorably to input from the plant kingdom. Hence the wisdom of making healing and balancing patterns available to us through plants. It's like a direct telephone linkup. From one direction you have the direct link with healing and balancing patterns as a result of the plant/central nervous system relationship. And from the other direction, because the disorder and dysfunction we experience first impact our bodies within the central nervous system, you have the early warning system. The two—the easy accessibility to the healing patterns held within plants and the early warning when the body dysfunctions—meet right at the central nervous system.

One result of disorder and dysfunction is that the corresponding electrical circuitry along the spinal column breaks, short-circuits. If nothing is done to rectify the situation, the related network of nerves receives weakened electrical impulses rather than the usual strong impulses. These weakened impulses travel through the nerves to their related areas of the body, especially the endocrine system. Immediately, there is physical weakness in that area which, if not addressed, results in illness or disease.

Another result causes what can best be described as "system overload." Disorder and dysfunction impact the central nervous system along the spinal column, causing the electrical circuitry to unbalance in such a way that the normal flow of electrical impulses dramatically increases. If the overload is not addressed, the body will physically respond with symptoms such as hyperactivity and twitching.

Because of the unique relationship between the plant kingdom and the central nervous system, flower essences, in a most efficient and dramatic manner, are able to reconnect the broken circuitry and rebalance the electrical overload along the spine. This, in turn, stops the weakening domino effect that ultimately leads to illness. If a person is too late in using the essences, and illness has already set in, the essences still reconnect and balance the circuitry and hold that balance while the body heals.

To help you with a basic understanding of the flower essences, I include a session on the subject from the *Perelandra Garden Workbook*. It was translated from the nature intelligence identified as the Overlighting Deva of Flower Essences. (A definition and explanation of devas is given later in this chapter.) Since this was part of the *Workbook*, the deva also relates flower essences to the co-creative energy gardening process that is described in the *Workbook*.

OVERLIGHTING DEVA OF FLOWER ESSENCES

I am part of what might be called "the healing devas," in that I am a part of a group of overlighting intelligences in nature who focus specifically on the various healing dynamics within and throughout the kingdoms of nature on planet Earth.

When the human soul chose to inspirit physical matter on the planet, we of nature consciously accepted a partnership with humans that related to the development of their physical form and

5

*all matters relating to what may best be described as the upkeep
and maintenance of that form in every way. In present-day terminol-
ogy, you may say that we have a "contractual agreement" with you
humans which was initiated prior to the human soul coming to the
planet and was fully activated the very instant the first souls entered
the planet's atmosphere. Nature has been completely at your disposal as you took on matter and developed your form. All that com-
prises human form is extracted from the three kingdoms of nature.*

*But form development and its maintenance through food, shelter,
and clothing is only a part of our agreement. In light of the universal law of horizontal healing, we also took on the responsibility to
balance the human form during times of dysfunction. So in these
areas we have overlighting healing devas who establish the patterns
in nature that respond to human form in healing ways and integrate
those patterns into the specific blueprint of individual plants,
animals, and minerals to be recognized, unlocked, and used appropriately by humans when needed. I will say to you now that
there is contained within nature a pattern of healing that responds
and relates to every specific dysfunction within mankind. It is an
ever-changing area of service, in that when specific diseases or dysfunctions are eliminated or released as part of the human experience, we devas who work in this area release the complementary healing pattern that has been held in custodianship within
nature. Conversely, when humans introduce and take on a new dysfunctional pattern, we respond immediately and infuse the appropriate balancing pattern within the blueprint of one or more
members of the kingdoms of nature.*

*What you call the "ecological problems" that you now face play
directly into the very area of service of which I have been speaking.
Simply put, we devas infuse the specific healing patterns in nature*

on their corresponding devic level. Those patterns are fully in-tegrated. As humans have disassociated themselves from the life balances of nature and moved into a consciousness of manipulating nature solely for their own ends, they have interfered with the successful fusion of that blueprint into its form. Consequently, the healing patterns, although still available, have become cloudy, un-focused, and less accessible to humans.

This brings me full circle to the enormous benefit that lies before those who consciously work to create a garden environment with the attitudes and intent as described in this book. [the Perelandra Garden Workbook] *By working the garden with a mind-set of co-creation rather than manipulation, one establishes an environment that is raised to a level of life above and beyond the ecological mes-ses surrounding it. This, in turn, allows for the healing patterns to be fully present and a part of the specific forms within the garden environment. The unlocking and understanding of those patterns will be clear and complete, and the appropriate form in which the patterns are released will be developed.*

It is not an exaggeration (although many will perceive it to be) to say that at some point in the future, the medical world will look to those who have established co-creative gardens to supply the pat-tern-infused solutions to be used within their own medical arena. These solutions will be recognized for their power, potency, and their ability to quickly get to the heart of a matter in order to return the human to balanced form. Do not underestimate the power and clarity that will be released from each co-creative garden as it estab-lishes its position of balance.

To address the issue of flower essences: We healing devas look to the plant kingdom as the primary recipients for the infusion of specific healing patterns. This is because the plant kingdom

7

responds to and resonates with the central nervous system in humans. All disorder and dysfunction are reflected in the nervous system, thus making accessible the problems to the plant kingdom. The scope of the nervous system in its various levels of function is no smaller than the universe itself. It is, in the body, the bridge that directly connects and fuses the soul to its form. Since the soul is linked to the universe at large, it is essential that the nervous system have, in form, the same capacity. Eventually, as soul and form balance, the nervous system will operate co-equally with the soul and translate all that is accessible to the soul into and through the body. There will be no separation between the human soul and his body.

As I stated earlier, humans borrowed from the three kingdoms in nature that which was needed for an appropriate form. For the central nervous system, he borrowed primarily from the plant kingdom. And, as I have also stated, it is the plant kingdom that we primarily utilize for infusing into the blueprint human healing patterns. As can easily be seen, it is most appropriate for mankind to look to the plant kingdom for these healing patterns.

It is especially appropriate for the individual and his family to draw from the garden environment flower essences from those specific plants that are useful in aiding and assisting their physical balance. Consider the following: It has been said that the co-creative garden environment shifts, balances, and enhances all that its energy envelops. This includes, of course, those individuals connected with the garden. As it reaches new levels of balance, the garden literally shifts and raises all that it touches to a level relative to that which it is now on itself. The process is continued, but in a different manner, when the food is eaten. Now those connected with the garden are being affected by its energy from without and within.

The physical form is receiving an enormous amount of input from this environment. Aside from the heart influence of the individual, it is the overriding healing impulse received by the body. To continue that impulse in the form of flower essences derived from the very environment of which I speak, is to move along the healing path without missing one step, one beat.

I bring another consideration to your attention. The individual is drawn at specific times throughout his life to live in the location that best serves his higher purpose. This is a truth. It does not discount human free will which allows him to override his inner knowing and establish himself in an environment based on willful desire. When the soul fuses into form it implants its own higher pattern into the nature energy in the body. At this time, like a computer readout, the individual takes on an awareness as to what environment he must be a part of in order for his higher purpose to be fully stabilized and supported in form. This includes the environmental conditions and the food he must have as well as the healing patterns contained in specific members of the nature kingdoms which must be made accessible to him. At various times you will observe individuals, or sense within yourself, a compulsive drive to move or change locations. This is that inner awareness coming into consciousness and, quite often, you will feel the healing power of the new location as soon as you enter it.

Do not misread what I am saying to mean that in a highly mobile society, the individual must strive for permanent roots or a series of long-term roots, or he will lose his opportunity to have needed access to important healing and stabilizing patterns. Remember that I said it is the higher purpose of the individual that fuses with nature, thus creating the awareness of appropriate environmental needs. If his higher purpose includes the scenario of many homes in quick succession, roots in many corners of the world, it will result in his desire to move around the planet in directions that place him in the environment that offers physical support and healing at specific times.

Now, people who are drawn to gardening respond to this inner impulse in a very concrete manner. Without realizing it, they create their garden from those plants and minerals that hold the very healing patterns they personally need. Don't forget that the garden is designed on the devic level in the spirit of full environmental balance. It is precisely that balanced energy to which his inner soul/form awareness resonates, not an ecologically imbalanced or damaged image of this balance. When they expand their gardening awareness to include the production of flower essences, they release from fully inspirited and empowered plants these healing patterns, thus enabling them to enter a new level of personal healing. This is, in fact, a continuation of that which was already begun when they responded to the inner soul/form resonance, settled in a specific location, and established their co-creative garden.

I cannot resist giving you a glimpse into the future, for you see, the relationship of humans to their movement around the planet is directly connected to this notion of their responding to environments that hold for them the very healing patterns they have needed. Humans are presently experiencing much mobility, a great desire to move around the planet, see the world, live in different cultures and environments. At this time in his evolution, it is important that he physically familiarize himself with the planet upon which he lives, for in the future, it will be the planet as a whole, not just one corner of it, that will be the focus of his higher soul patterns and the support for his physical vehicle. Humans are rapidly moving into an era of global consciousness. The drive to be physically present in many different countries and cultures is preparing him for this shift, not just intellectually and emotionally, but physically and spiritually as well. As he travels, his body experiences and responds to new natural patterns, not just cultural patterns. This exposure opens him to the healing patterns needed in order to expand his physical body balance so that it can fully support the expansion of his awareness of himself and the world in which he lives.

You will note that the emphasis in the present time is one of physical movement around the planet. But the population as a whole is moving into a new era in which movement around the planet will be primarily accomplished on the inner levels through the development and use of the sixth sense. The physical bridge for this era is already being established through the technology of electronics and computers. These technologies are beginning to supply, through the use of physical form, what will be accomplished in the future through the use of the sixth sense. Countries are linking in ways that were never before imagined. Individuals have instantaneous connection and communication with others in areas that used to take days of utilizing the best, most efficient transportation modes to reach. Many have noted that the world is becoming smaller, as they say. Well, it is not really becoming smaller, it is becoming whole.

Once this shift occurs and humans have instant communication through the sixth sense with anyone anywhere on the planet, the need to physically travel will no longer exist. You will see humans physically a part of one environment while at the same time experiencing total access to the rest of the planet.

This will create a change in how the human relates to the environment for physical support and healing. Remember that now the fusion of the higher purpose into form is still, for all intents and purposes, regional. It requires that the individual enter and experience a specific environment for support and healing. In the future, the higher purpose will be global yet, at the same time, not require physical presence in every environment. At that time, the individual will be drawn back into establishing stable, long-term roots in an area that gives him his basic, natural support. In the beginning, he will need to pull to him the elements of nature from outside areas that will round out the support for his new global balance. It is quite conceivable that the primary source of global balance will not come in the form of imported food but rather in the form of flower essences made from ecologically balanced, co-creative gardens throughout the world. The high quality of nature support derived from the plant essences resonating to the greater-sensitized human central nervous system will be the most desired form of global natural interchange. And the multitude of co-creative gardens then in existence will link in a new way and respond in global service to human healing.

In a session I had in 1984 with a consciousness known to me as Universal Light, flower essences were directly linked to the universal principle called "horizontal healing." In a nutshell, horizontal healing means that for the most comprehensive and efficient healing, one should seek what he needs for healing from within the same dimension as the problem being manifested. That is, aspects from the physical world being used to heal problems manifesting within the physical body. Emotional problems being addressed from the level of emotions. Mental problems from the mental. Spiritual from the level of the spiritual. Like healing like. More often than not, any individual problem manifests on all of these levels simultaneously. The principle of horizontal healing encourages us to look for full healing from input on all those levels, each input directly related to how the problem is manifesting on its specific level. According to this principle, one will not achieve full healing of a problem manifesting on all four levels by addressing, for example, just the physical issues or just the emotional issues.

UNIVERSAL LIGHT

The effect of the flower essences on form (we use "form" to indicate all form, not just human) is directly related to a universal principle: the healing process that occurs on the horizontal level. Although we may not have flower essences per se on other levels of reality, in other corners of this universe, the principle of horizontal movement, or connection, within the same level of reality remains.

To explain: Flower essences are form (flowers) released into another substance which is also form (water) and then given for the healing and balancing of form within a human, an animal, another plant, or even a rock. There is a strong healing quality between like and like. Edward Bach [London physician and developer of the Bach Flower Essences in the early 1930s] *understood this when he shifted from the traditional homeopathic concept (of negative and positive — in other words, two negatives creating a positive) to that of the flower essences (of two positives, of like connecting to like). On a personality level, one finds a healing experience when he relates to a person of like mind and feels, during this communication or interchange, a sense of ease, balance, healing, and understanding. Similarly, the flower essences relate to the body or to form — one might say they are of like mind; they are horizontally connected and related.*

13

Many flower essence practitioners and many people who use flower essences feel that the essences are successful because they respond to the soul, respond beyond the level of form. To put it bluntly, this is not true. Man understands neither the level of form nor the expansiveness within his own level. Flower essences respond from the level of form to the level of form and are highly successful for that reason. The same holds true in any natural healing process throughout the history of herbs, plants, and healing. The mountain doctor or mountain woman who heals through the use of plants, the witch doctor in Africa who heals through the use of plants and minerals, and the Indian who uses plants, minerals, and crystals have all touched into their "brothers" (all of which are form). They have found a friend of like mind who is able and eager to come to and into them for the purpose of healing, balancing, and reestablishing stability.

There are many hundreds of flower essences now being produced by a number of people. I am familiar with and have used the Bach Flower Essences (produced in England) and the FES Flower Essences (produced by the Flower Essence Society in California). I am including in *Bibliography and Resources* their names and addresses. I encourage you to write for information to these people and others who may attract your attention and to follow your own sense of good judgment and intuition as to which flower essences are for you. However, in this book I will explain flower essences by presenting the essences I know best—the Perelandra Rose Essences and the Perelandra Garden Essences.

A LITTLE ABOUT PERELANDRA

Perelandra is both home for Clarence and me and a nature research center. It consists of forty-five acres of mostly woods in the foothills of the Blue Ridge Mountains in Virginia. The nature research and development has been going on since 1976, when I opened to and dedicated myself to learning about nature in new ways from nature itself. I began working with nature intelligences in a coordinated, co-creative, and educational effort which has resulted in understanding and demonstrating a new approach to ecological balance.

The primary focus of my work has been the one-hundred-foot-diameter circular garden where I receive from nature the information and direction I need to create an all-inclusive garden environment based on the principles of energy in balance. For example, we do not attempt to repel insects, but rather we focus on creating a balanced environment that calls to it and fully supports a complete and appropriate population of insects. In turn, the insects relate to the garden's plant life in a light and nondestructive manner.

From this kind of work has developed a new method of gardening I call "co-creative energy gardening." Briefly, this is a method of gardening in partnership with the nature intelligences that emphasizes balance and teamwork. The balance is a result of concentrating on the laws of the life energy behind form. The teamwork is established between the individual and the intelligent levels inherent in nature. (Information about this work is described in two books: *Behaving As If the God In All Life Mattered:*

15

A New Age Ecology and the *Perelandra Garden Workbook: A Complete Guide to Gardening with Nature Intelligences*. Both are listed on the Perelandra order form which is included in the back of the book.)

The foundation of the work going on at Perelandra, as I have indicated, comes from nature intelligences, a collective term I use for devas and nature spirits. My work with flower essences has also been directed from these levels. Therefore, it would be helpful if I gave you an idea of who and what these intelligences are.

"Deva" is a sanskrit word used to describe the intelligent level of consciousness within nature that functions in an architectural mode within all that is of form and also serves as the organizer of all that is a part of each form. This means that if I should want to understand or change something in the botanical makeup of a plant species, I would consult with the deva of that species for clarification regarding my specific questions and for advice as to whether my change is viable or ecological. The deva of each type of plant holds the architectural blueprints of that plant and has the power to change the blueprints at any time.

"Nature spirit" refers to the intelligent level of consciousness within nature that works in partnership with the devic level and is responsible for the fusing and maintaining of energy to appropriate form. They tend to the shifting of an energy reality that has been formulated on the devic level and assist the translation of that reality from a dynamic of energy to form. They also function in a custodial capacity with all that is of form on the planet.

Flower essences, their development, and their uses have been a natural outgrowth of the work being done in the Perelandra garden. They are considered part of its harvest. The Perelandra Rose Essences were developed beginning in 1984 from eight specific

16

rose bushes that are a part of the outermost ring of roses in the garden. The Perelandra Garden Essences were developed in 1986 as a result of my asking the Overlighting Deva of Flower Essences the question: "Using the makeup of the Perelandra garden as your base, what vegetables, herbs, and flowers would you choose to be made into flower essences that would best address the issues people face today?" I was given a list of eighteen plants which I quickly produced as the Perelandra Garden Essences.

The various principles of energy and balance that have been demonstrated so successfully in the garden have been extended to the Perelandra Rose and Garden Essences. So included in this book, in order to understand the essences, is information on various principles of energy, balance, and form and the resulting processes that have incorporated them.

2

How the Perelandra Flower Essences Are Made

ONE WAY TO DISPEL the mystique surrounding flower essences is to tell you how they are made. Well, at least I can tell you precisely how the Perelandra essences are made. The physical process is generally the same all over. Interspersed throughout the following directions are the original explanatory comments given me from the Deva of Flower Essences so that I could understand why I do what I do.

DIRECTIONS FOR CO-CREATIVE
FLOWER ESSENCE PREPARATION

TOOLS AND INGREDIENTS:
You'll need: scissors, long tweezers, 2-qt. clear glass batter bowl (with handle), glass saucer or plate, untreated or distilled water, quart canning jars and lids, brandy.

Best time for selecting flowers: 8 a.m.-10:30 a.m.

Choose flowers that are about one day from being fully open.

Deva of Flower Essences: *At this time you have the flower on the upswing in energy and just prior to releasing its full potency to the environment. By harvesting the flower at this stage, you will allow it to release its full potency to the water instead of the environment.*

I clean with hot, soapy water all utensils (including scissors and tweezers), the bowl and the saucer or plate, and two quart canning jars and lids. I don't touch the inside surface of the bowl or jars after washing. This will assure that my personal energy will not commingle with the essence tincture.

1. I connect with the Deva of Flower Essences to determine how many flowers are needed to convert one quart of water to full-essence solution. Usually this will be just one to five flowers, depending mostly on size. With tiny flowers, more tend to be needed. Ninety-five percent of the time I will be working only with the flower of the plant. If I sense differently, I ask the deva if this is one of the times when I'm to use the plant's leaves.

2. I concentrate on gathering the flowers for one essence at a time. The flowers are cut without my touching or sniffing them so that the energy is not altered or dispersed. They are caught on the glass saucer as I cut, if it is difficult to get a long enough stem for holding.

3. In my work area, I remove the petals with scissors or tweezers (whatever method is most efficient without touching the petals with my fingers), allowing the petals to fall onto the glass saucer.

4. The large batter bowl is filled with one quart of untreated or distilled water.

5. Using the tweezers, lift the petals one by one from the glass saucer, shaking off all stamens, and place them in the bowl of water so that each petal touches the water surface. By the way, flower petals float.

6. I place the bowl, uncovered, in a sunny spot in the garden on a table I've set up for this.

Deva of Flower Essences: *The interaction of the sun's energy directly on the petals and water plays an important part in the essence-making process. Since sun is important, I suggest that essences be made on a sunny day!*

If I am making more than one flower essence that day, I then collect the flowers for the next one, prepare it, place it into the bowl of water, and place it on the table in the sun, leaving plenty of room between bowls. I repeat this until all the prepared bowls are in the sun. I usually don't make more than four different essences on any given day.

7. At this point in the process, I open to and connect with the nature spirit who works with me in the essence-making process. Without touching the bowl, I place my open hands next to each side of it (palms up, as if I were cupping it) and ask the nature spirit to release the healing and balancing pattern of the petals in full potency to the water. I allow about fifteen seconds for the process to complete before removing my hands. I repeat this process for each bowl. Every time, I have felt the power and energy being released from the petals. It feels like the energy moves through the water and hits my hands.

Deva of Flower Essences: *The release is done etherically, then grounded into the water form by the interaction with the sun. The release of the healing pattern by the nature spirit will occur instantly. The grounding process takes:*

3 hrs. — full sunny day

4 hrs. — partly sunny day

6 hrs. — cloudy day (Avoid if possible.)

Although the nature spirit level can ground energy into form instantly, it is preferable, in this case, that the seating of the essence into form be done in "form timing" not "energy timing." The grounding via form timing will more fully resonate horizontally to other form for healing.

Note: If bugs fall into the water, a one-layer covering of white gauze will protect the water without interfering with the sun's interaction with the water and petals. No extra time need be added onto the grounding process.

(In the beginning, I thought I would have a bug problem. We have countless squads of them in the garden, and I assumed at least a squad or two would nose-dive into these inviting bowls of floating flowers. So I armed myself with a bunch of white gauze. And the odd thing is, I've never used it. For whatever reason, bugs simply steer clear of the bowls. I like to think it has something to do with the quality of the essence-making process being used!)

8. After the allotted time, I bring the glass bowls, making sure to touch only the handle or the outside of the bowl, back to the work area. I'm careful to place them so that they don't touch.

With *clean* tweezers, I remove the petals from the first bowl. It does not affect the potency or clarity of the essence if metal or plastic touches or is immersed into the solution as long as they are clean.

9. I fill two quart canning jars to just under the 16-ounce mark with brandy. The ratio of brandy to flower essence is 40 percent brandy to 60 percent solution, or 50-50 percent. There should not be more than 50 percent brandy. The brandy is used as a preservative. In simple terms, it keeps slimy green things from growing in the essence tincture. With the proper amount of brandy preservative, the essences may be stored indefinitely at room temperature.

10. I fill the remainder of each jar (up to the 1-quart mark) with the flower essence solution. Then I securely screw on clean lids and bands and label the jar with the essence name and the date it was made.

11. I repeat steps 8 through 10 for each essence I'm making.

12. I place the quart jars of preserved and sealed essence in the center of the Perelandra garden for a final shift and stabilizing process. There, each jar is set inside a copper genesa crystal (an antenna-like form that draws to it life energy, then cleanses it, and shifts it up "a spiral") and enhanced with tensor energy (commonly known as "pyramid energy") and clear quartz and topaz energy. All parts—the flower essence and brandy tincture, and tensor and mineral energy—are fully coalesced into one stable, fully balanced unit. Since this is an energy step, sunshine is not necessary. I leave the jars in the genesa crystal for one hour. I've been advised not to place more than eight jars at a time in our two-foot-diameter genesa crystal.

The above steps may be used for making your own flower essences. If you would like to understand more about creating a balanced nature environment in cooperation with the intelligences of nature from which to harvest the flowers for your essences, I suggest the *Perelandra Garden Workbook*. Also, it will give you a clear idea of how to go about enlisting the aid of nature spirits in the essence-making process. But if you would like to just go ahead and make some essences using the above steps and with the aid of the nature spirit level without bothering with the *Workbook*, there's really a way you can do this. It's not some great and difficult mystery. Just set yourself up according to the steps, and when it comes time to work with nature spirits, simply request their assistance and let them know what precisely you wish them to do. Then proceed forward in trust. I hate to say it's that easy, but in actuality, it is that easy. You just need to be clear and precise. Don't be afraid to express yourself aloud – this little trick will assist you in getting your thoughts about the matter clear and concise.

If you make your own essences, at this point you are faced with quart jars of the stuff. A quart of solution will last you and your loved ones for approximately three to five generations. I offer several hints from a seasoned flower essence practitioner – me.

I suggest you buy from the local pharmacy a one-half-ounce dropper bottle for each different flower essence you've made. Transfer tincture into these bottles, label them, and use them for your day-to-day needs. That way, if you contaminate the tincture in any way, you can pour it out, clean the bottle, and refill it from your quart stock. Since you are using the flower essences only a drop at a time, it is most unwieldy to try to use them directly from the quart jar, and in the case of contamination (something children and animals are especially gifted at doing by touching the droppers with their tongues), you won't lose the entire quart solution.

The easiest way that I have found to transfer the solution is with a kitchen baster. I have been told that it is important to store the tincture in glass containers, but it is okay to transfer the tincture from container to container using clean plastic or metal utensils. It was also suggested to me in the original instructions that for the transfer of the tincture to small bottles, the same spirit of cleanliness and care not to contaminate either human to essence, or essence to essence, be continued.

For the entire set of utensils, bowls, plates, and jars I use in the flower essence process, I make it a point to use them for this only. I do not use the batter bowl in the kitchen or the baster for that night's turkey.

The flower essences you purchase in sets of small bottles (dram or half-ounce) are diluted once again. For the Perelandra essences, a one-half-ounce dropper bottle is filled with brandy (distilled white vinegar for those who are allergic to brandy), and ten drops of the quart-jar essence tincture are added. This is considered a concentrate of the flower essence and labeled as such. Ten drops sound outrageous – especially since we live in an age when such drastic, hard-hitting things are done to us in the name of health. The no-pain-no-gain mentality. But our electrical system operates completely and efficiently with the lightest of touches – feather touch. To illustrate the point even further, at the time of use, you may choose to dilute them further by putting a few drops of each essence in four ounces of water. Full essence power is still maintained.

OVERLIGHTING DEVA OF FLOWER ESSENCES

In order to understand what Machaelle refers to as "the lightest of touches," let us add some additional insight. We refer you back to the principle of horizontal healing—like healing like. The vibratory healing pattern that is released from the flower petal to the water is on the electrical level. We of the devic level could have chosen for that pattern to release into the water on any vibratory level as long as it related directly to form, to the physical reality of all life on planet Earth. We chose the electrical level for two reasons: One, the most efficient level in which to address imbalance in the form is on the electrical level. In the human body, the central nervous system with its network of nerves allows instantaneous access to the body as a whole. In essence, a complete system or network was already in place and, to be frank, could not have been more potentially efficient. Two, there are many more people inhabiting the planet than there are numbers of individual flowers. Sheer logistics became a consideration in the original decisions on the method of imprinting human healing patterns through the vehicle of plant flowers. If we were to release the pattern on a purely physical vibratory level, you would need to use one flower per dose of essence. Considering the present population, it would not take very long to eradicate plant life on the planet once the idea of flower essences caught on. Due to its properties, the electrical vibratory level allows the pattern to infuse into a water solution at such a high concentration that the essence may be diluted many times over in order to be made available to the population as a whole without damaging the ecological balance of the planet.

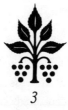

3

Definitions

THE INFORMATION SUPPLIED to you by the definitions of flower essences is as vital to the healing and balancing process as the physical support they give to the body. Essences offer a two-prong attack in that they not only physically reconnect, balance, and support you electrically, but they also give you insight into what is causing the problem. We all have stressful and difficult life experiences. What the flower essences tell us is which of those experiences at any given time is so intense that we are responding by short-circuiting or overloading.

Definitions are the identification of the specific healing pattern that has been released from the flower into the water. They are obtained in a number of ways — most of them not traditional. It is my understanding that Edward Bach, the London physician who developed the first modern set of flower essences in the 1930s, had the ability to place himself in extreme states of emotional and physical distress. Then he walked through the countryside of England touching different flowers, plants, and trees one at a time until he experienced relief and balancing. That gave him the clue as to what the specific plant addressed. He then verified this information by using them accordingly on his patients and keeping detailed records of the results. His experience combined with their experience became the basis for the Bach Flower Essence definitions.

Others who have since developed additional flower essences have used intuition and/or channeling combined with personal experience with the essence, as well as outside verification from others' experience to arrive at specific definitions. Sometimes the definitions are lengthy, sometimes quite short. Often they are given as simply a guidepost for the users to add to according to their personal experience.

With the Perelandra Rose and Garden Essences, I got the definitions by directly contacting the Deva of Flower Essences along with the deva of the plant involved and learned what the specific pattern is dealing with. I then watched how the essences held up in testing with myself and others in light of these definitions for verification that what I received was accurate.

A personal note here. I do not channel. The devas do not take over my physical being nor do they control my voice. I do what I call "translation." I am in full control of my consciousness. I connect with specific devas and nature spirits in much the same manner as two people connected via a phone line. Information is given me in the form of energy. My job as translator is to assign to specific impulses of energy the word that most fully carries the intent of the energy I was given. To understand this process more easily, just think of the job of the United Nations' interpreters. They don't go into a trance state. They develop the art of focused listening and the ability to translate intent, thought, expression, and concept from one language pattern to another. If you take away the audible sound and have only the projection to the translator of the energy behind the sound, you have an idea of what I receive: communication in the form of energy. I just translate that communication into the form of words that are faithful to the intent and expression of the energy I "hear." And very like the U.N. interpreter, I am only as good at this as my innate ability combined with training, discipline, care, and a lot of years of practice.

To give you an idea of how flower essence definitions can sound, I am including the Perelandra definitions for both the Garden Essences and the Rose Essences sets. Their intent and approach to health and dysfunction are quite different. The name of the essence is the name of the plant from which it was made. The definition is the actual information I received from the devic level.

PERELANDRA GARDEN ESSENCES

BROCCOLI: Power. Several of these flower essences [the Perelandra Garden Essences] will deal with the state of power. It is one of the most sought-after states today and perhaps the least understood. Consequently, individuals who relinquish their personal infinite power take on the trappings of surface finite power in their misguided attempts to rediscover and reconnect with their infinite power. Infinite power is a complex issue in that it connotes balance on all levels in every way. Therefore, you will see coming to the foreground, in the area of flower essences, those flowers that address various avenues and aspects of power.

The balancing pattern contained in broccoli focuses on the power balance that must be maintained when the individual perceives himself to be under siege on any or all of the four levels of his being. (By levels, we mean the physical, emotional, mental, and spiritual or universal.) [Referred to from here on as "p.e.m.s."] The source of the siege is perceived to be outside rather than within. The potential here is for a strong reaction of self-protection. In an attempt to isolate and contain the level from which the threat seems to be occurring, there is a sudden closing down and detachment from any or all of the four levels. This renders the individual powerless, for he has scattered himself to the four winds. The essence of broccoli stabilizes the body/soul unit during this intense time, thus enabling confrontation of the perceived siege as a fully functioning and balanced body/soul unit. Broccoli Essence will be especially useful to those going through deep emotional wrenching such as separation or divorce, those suffering from hallucinations or mental illness that includes hallucinations as part of its pattern, and those experiencing what are perceived to be frightening sixth-sense incidents, experience, or expansions.

CAULIFLOWER: In the future, the essence of cauliflower will be known as "the birth essence." Whereas the Perelandra Rose Essences deal with transition and transformation on all levels throughout one's life and death process, the essence of cauliflower holds the stabilizing patterns specifically for the experience of birth. Many of the dysfunctional patterns an individual experiences throughout his entire life cycle are fused into the body and soul during the process of birth. These patterns are a result of the body/soul balance being thrown off center due to the child's refusal to maintain conscious awareness during birth. The essence of cauliflower supports and stabilizes the awareness of both the higher, expanded soul and the conscious child-soul as the two move through birth. With these two levels stabilized in process, the body/soul unit of the child maintains its balance, thus eliminating instances of imbalance that crystallize into the child's body as dysfunctional patterns.

The Cauliflower Essence will not prevent the child from experiencing the kind of birth that is keyed into the evolutionary pattern from its soul level. It will, however, assist his ability to maintain full awareness and to focus on purpose as he moves through the birth.

THE CAULIFLOWER ESSENCE BIRTH-STABILIZING PROCESS: The mother should begin this support of the child's process as soon as contractions begin. One or two drops of Cauliflower Essence taken every two hours will provide the necessary internal environment for the child. By concentrating her attention on the baby at the time she is administering the drops to herself, the mother will "telegraph" the vibration of the essence directly to the child. If possible, continue the two-hour rhythm right up to birth. At the first opportunity after birth, place one drop of Cauliflower Essence directly on the lips of the newborn child and another drop two hours after birth. (Two drops of essence concentrate may be diluted in eight ounces of water. Two drops of this solution placed on the baby's lips will be tasteless.) Administer one drop concentrate or two drops water solution each morning for the next two days. This will conclude the Cauliflower Essence stabilizing process.

[NOTE: It may become necessary to support the baby with follow-up essences after the process period is complete. By maintaining conscious awareness during birth, babies seem to maintain one foot in the child-body plane and the other foot in the soul plane, with birth as the bridge. The result is that they move through birth with a strong sense of purpose and deliberation,

31

and afterwards may need essence support as they go through a three-month period of integration. It is advisable to test (to be explained later) the child after the birth-stabilizing process is complete to see if further essences are needed and, if so, to maintain an essence vigilance until the child tests as fully stabilized. This may take any time up to three months.

Also, adults are testing a need for Cauliflower Essence. At the appropriate time, they can connect with the same kind of body/soul balance that the newborns are establishing during the Cauliflower birth process. Cauliflower Essence supports this connection in the adult.

More information on Cauliflower Essence is included in Chapter 8.]

CELERY: Restores the balance of the immune system during times when the system is being overworked or stressed. This essence is particularly helpful during long-term illnesses caused by viral or bacterial infections that overpower and can eventually break down the immune system altogether. The essence of celery holds the balancing support for the immune system during such times.

CHIVES: Power. Chives Essence reestablishes the power one has when the internal male/female dynamics are balanced and the individual is functioning in a state of awareness within this balance. Although the herbal essence of chives would seem to indicate a leaning toward the masculine dynamic, the flower essence holds the pattern for balance between the two, no matter which is predominant at any given time.

COMFREY: The essence of comfrey repairs higher vibrational soul damage that may be the result of this or another lifetime. It will sometimes be used in combination with other flower essences that respond more directly to the cause(s) of the damage.

CORN: Traditionally corn has been used for enhancing the spiritualization of Earth and human alike. Specifically, the essence of corn stabilizes the body/soul fusion of an individual during times of spiritual or universal expansion. Rather than focusing on the expansive soul seeking to move through the finite body, Corn Essence balances the individual during those times his conscious being (which is fully of the Earth, responding to an inner yearning) reaches up and out into that vast universal expansion. Quite often, the individual responds to his yearnings by releasing himself from his physical reality and jettisoning into the universe. This vastly limits the usefulness of the experience in his daily physical reality. Corn Essence assists the individual in holding that body/soul fusion, thus allowing him to translate the universal experience into useful, pertinent understanding and action.

CUCUMBER: The essence of cucumber is to be used to rebalance the individual during times of depression. By this, we mean those times when one feels completely detached from his life and perceives it to be a picture show playing out in front of him, but not involving him. The individual has little or no desire to reenter the picture. Cucumber Essence strengthens the psyche, which allows the individual to move from a state of depression to a vital, positive reattachment to his life.

DILL: Power. Dill Essence is very useful to those who have released their personal power to others and as a result live through their day-to-day routine having taken on the attitude of the victim. It assists the individual in reclaiming balance in the area of personal power, thus resulting in a shift in his relationship with those around him.

NASTURTIUM: Vital life energy on the physical level. When an individual is working predominantly from his head, his physical body will not only atrophy within the muscle structure but in the area of vital life energy as well. This energy, as a dynamic, is directly connected to the muscle structure. Nasturtium Essence assists in keeping that connection and revitalizing the energy itself, when necessary. It has a grounding effect within the individual in that it maintains life vitality in the physical, especially at times when the focus and power on the mental level are pulling that energy to the mental processes.

OKRA: There are those, and I refer to quite a large group of people, who insist on seeing or translating their reality in the worst possible light. Neither depressed, for they express strong energy, nor just angry, these are people who have lost the ability to perceive beauty and joy on all levels. Okra Essence restores this ability. Now, it may sound to be a "frivolous" essence — one given to a grumpy uncle — but these people live in such an all-encompassing atmosphere of gloom and doom that their attitudes challenge their physical health and well-being. Also, they create such a strong negative environment that they draw to them other negativities that exist beyond their immediate environment. Like attracting like. Eventually they create islands of powerful negative forces that dot the surface of the earth. Although not evil, these people have lost the ability to see the positive.

SALVIA: Emotional stability during times of extreme stress. Salvia Essence is very helpful when an individual is plummeted into an extreme, intense, emergency situation, either with himself or someone close, such as sudden injury, an automobile accident, a nuclear accident, or the diagnosis of serious illness—those times when one becomes emotionally broadsided and feels there is nowhere to turn. This essence restores emotional stability which, in turn, allows the individual to think and function in balance as he moves through the most extreme times.

SNAP PEA (GARDEN PEA): The snap pea is a fairly recent development in the garden pea family, but it carries the balancing pattern that is a part of the overall family vibration. We refer to the situation of frightening, tension-provoking dreams—nightmares. It is especially effective with children and those of child-like minds, such as the mentally or emotionally impaired. The essence of snap pea assists the individual with the translation of experience into positive, understandable process. If an individual is prone to frightening dreams, it is because he has not developed an alternative positive pattern for translating stress or fear. He has only this one avenue. Now, we do not include the occasional frightening dream that all experience from time to time. Rather, we refer to a frequent pattern of nightmares. Snap Pea Essence (or any Garden Pea Essence) supports the individual and allows him to develop alternative, less frightening ways of expressing emotion or experience.

Because of the support dynamic of this essence, it can also be given to someone who doesn't have frequent nightmares but who has just experienced one particularly powerful nightmare and is having difficulty pulling out of it. Snap Pea Essence supports and enhances the ability to detach from frightening internal experience.

SUMMER SQUASH (YELLOW): Courage. Whereas the Peace Essence in the Perelandra Rose Essence set pertains to the alignment of the individual to the dynamic of universal courage during times of transition and transformation, the courage of the Summer Squash Essence stabilizes the person who experiences fear and resistance when faced with his daily routine. The stability given by this essence during such times will restore the sense of calm courage needed to move forward through the day. Especially helpful to those suffering from shyness or phobias.

SWEET BELL PEPPER (GREEN): Inner peace. Sweet Bell Pepper Essence restores inner balance to the individual who lives and works in a stressful environment. It helps the person move through stressful situations with clarity and inner calm. In today's society, one could say, "Who doesn't have a stressful life?" Humans are presently seeking to understand and integrate ways that will enable them to live a hectic, fast-paced lifestyle while remaining healthy and in balance. Sweet Bell Pepper Essence will greatly facilitate this process, and a single drop in the morning can be as much a part of the daily routine to release stress as exercising and proper diet. This essence both stabilizes the body/soul balance during stressful situations and restores that balance should a situation throw it off. In short, it may be taken as part of the daily routine, before a specific situation that is perceived to be stressful, or after an experience should the individual be caught off guard.

TOMATO: Cleansing. Tomato Essence is helpful when infection or disease have become seated in the body. It is particularly useful when the endocrine system is involved. This essence both stabilizes the areas of imbalance and assists the body in shattering and throwing off that which is causing the infection or disease. We use the word "shattering" deliberately, because the Tomato Essence does indeed respond swiftly in the body and in a manner that appears, or may even feel, to be shattering. If the immune system has been weakened by the situation, one may need to take Celery Essence in combination with Tomato Essence.

Do not overlook this essence for the small scrape or wound that may potentially develop into a minor infection. It will be useful at these times, as well, and could be considered as essential a part of your home first-aid as the Band-Aid. It may be taken orally or sprayed directly on a cut or scrape, with equal effectiveness.

YELLOW YARROW: Yarrow as a flower essence has been used for protection on the emotional level during times of vulnerability caused by spiritual and psychological growth process. Yellow Yarrow Essence, in particular, is helpful during these times in that it not only protects one from outside influence during periods of emotional vulnerability, but it supports the individual in a way that allows him to soften on all levels so that the integration of his shifts can occur more easily. It protects and at the same time returns one to a state of softness, gentleness. This essence is especially effective for those who respond to their times of vulnerability by throwing up a wall—a wall that impedes their integration process.

ZINNIA: Restores the individual's sense of playfulness, laughter, and joy. Zinnia Essence assists in achieving a balanced and healthful sense of priority while allowing the letting go of those things that need not matter quite so much. It reminds the individual of the balance of a child's laughter and joy, and helps him contact the child within for his balance.

ZUCCHINI: Physical strength. The Zucchini Essence is especially helpful during times of convalescence after childbirth, illness, or surgery, when the body is working to restore physical vitality. It may be taken during an illness as well, for the essence will assist the individual in maintaining as much of his physical strength as possible while going through the illness process.

PERELANDRA ROSE ESSENCES

The Rose Essences address the issue of the full internal process required during day-to-day change. Whereas the Garden Essences deal with specific issues, the Rose Essences deal with the process of everyday change no matter what the issue. There are eight essences in the set, each addressing a specific facet in this change process, from beginning to end.

Since the Rose Essences were developed, people have expressed interest in knowing the color of each rose variety used. I include this information after each name.

GRUSS AN AACHEN: (salmon-shaded pink) Gruss an Aachen stabilizes the body and soul on all levels [p.e.m.s.] while the individual moves forward in evolutionary process. Gruss an Aachen supports and holds the body/soul unit while one enters and moves through an evolutionary stage which can bring up intense challenges and fears. After testing [see chapter on kinesiology], registering a positive for Gruss an Aachen would signify that one is experiencing not a body/soul-threatening situation but movement along his evolutionary path which feels unfamiliar to him. Its unknown direction is bringing up sensations of fear, shock, and trauma on some or all of the p.e.m.s. levels. Gruss an Aachen calms these sensations and stabilizes the body/soul as a unit, giving the individual confidence and support as he moves forward. Since Gruss an Aachen may need to be administered through a large part (or even all) of the change process, do not be surprised if its use is indicated for several weeks or months. The main characteristic here is the conscious, forward motion of the body and soul as a unit, rather than an inner movement of the soul to which the body unconsciously reacts. For a while, each individual will need to go through a period of learning, becoming acquainted with and adjusting to this new dynamic of the soul and body consciously moving forward as a unit. In practice, Gruss an Aachen will often be combined with another Rose or Garden Essence — the former functioning as the supporter and the latter responding to the specific dynamics of the particular forward movement. Gruss an Aachen's need will be especially evident during the major transitions of birth and death.

PEACE: (yellow edged in pink) Courage. Do not let its name confuse you, for this essence deals directly with the dynamic of courage, not peace! Whereas Gruss an Aachen stabilizes and supports the body/soul unit during change and growth, Peace opens to the individual that inner courage which all possess on the highest and clearest of soul levels. This dynamic of courage is within all individuals and is drawn from continuously on an unconscious level. Once the body and soul begin to function together as a conscious unit, the individual may need to be reminded from time to time that this inner courage, connected with universal courage, is there for the asking and the taking. Peace aligns the individual to his own momentum to move forward, but it is the courage aligned to the larger universal dynamic and from deep within each soul that gives momentum to the soul and moves the universe forward.

ECLIPSE: (golden) Acceptance and insight. Eclipse rounds out the picture of change and growth. It carries the dynamic of acceptance, of getting out of one's own way, of gentle resignation, as well as appreciation of one's inner knowing. Related to this is the dynamic of insight: Since the body and soul are functioning as a unit, one cannot continue to move forward in a state of blind acceptance or resignation. The functioning of the body and soul as a consciously cooperating unit enables the mind to receive the soul's insight, and one's evolutionary path becomes stronger, clearer, more direct and grounded. Eclipse supports the mechanism between the body and soul through which the body receives soul input and insight. The related essences indicate the emotional dynamics that can rise up to distort, clog, or complicate this particular body/soul connection. Thus, Eclipse may be needed during the latter stages of evolutionary process when the body/soul insight mechanism is more likely to be functioning. Eclipse will not bypass or override an individual's timing. He will not suddenly be confronted by an insight with which he is not ready to deal. Eclipse enhances an individual's understanding of his own timing and process.

ORANGE RUFFLES: (orange, shaded from brilliant orange to saffron yellow) Receptivity. An individual moving forward as a conscious body/soul unit will experience receptivity in a new way. This essence stabilizes the individual on all p.e.m.s. levels as the soul infusion (the seating of the soul into the body) encourages the expansion of the parameters of the individual's sensory system. Orange Ruffles helps stabilize the individual as his sensory system expands so that he may function with new sensitivity to each of the five physical senses. This essence will not cause the expansion of an individual's sensory system. It will, however, stabilize the individual as he moves through the shift from one level of sensory functioning to another. Such a shift may be the sole purpose of an evolutionary step, or it may be in conjunction with an expansion requiring the individual to become more receptive in order to fully perceive a larger process.

AMBASSADOR: (soft orange-red) Pattern. Ambassador has to do with the relationship of the part to the whole: how a movement forward fits into the whole of the individual's life, the whole of the situation and/or environment around him, and eventually the whole of the planet and universe. This essence also relates to the dynamic of purpose, for when one is ready to consciously move forward, his momentum and desire are frequently drawn from a sense of purpose. However, a movement forward may create such challenge in an individual that his reaction eventually blocks his ability to grasp purpose, and may result in the draining of the energy needed to sustain him as he moves through a specific process. By stabilizing him on all p.e.m.s. levels, Ambassador aids by shifting the blocks to a position of balance, thus allowing the individual to receive purpose and see how the pattern of his movement fits into the larger patterns of the whole. To sum up, Ambassador relates to pattern, purpose, and vitality on all levels.

NYMPHENBURG: (apricot buds, with salmon-pink flowers shaded in orange, pink, and yellow) Strength. Nymphenburg enhances the strength created by a balanced body/soul fusion. There is an energy created when the body fully receives the soul within its own form which can best be described as an energy of strength. Nymphenburg facilitates and stabilizes that body/soul fusion. If the brain were used to symbolize this phenomenon, one could say the left brain represents the body, the right brain represents the soul, and the midbrain contains within itself the energy that connects the two. The balance between the two halves creates an even stronger energy in the midbrain which, in turn, further stabilizes that balance. Returning to the individual: When someone takes on an evolutionary move, the challenge of that move may threaten or upset the body/soul balance, thus diminishing the power of the very energy that stabilizes the balance. Nymphenburg supports and holds that strength, which facilitates the individual's ability to regain the balance of his body/soul fusion. In conscious evolutionary processes, maintaining this balance is essential.

WHITE LIGHTNIN': (pure white with occasional faint pink blush) Synchronized movement. White Lightnin' relates to the phenomenon of synchronized movement, which in conscious evolutionary progression is experienced in depth and breadth on all p.e.m.s. levels. Ideally, shifts corresponding to a specific progression move in concert with one another, and movement on individual levels is supportive of movement of the whole, i.e., the person's shift and growth on all the p.e.m.s. levels. Therefore, maintaining the timing and shifting on all these levels is essential to the stability of the shift as a whole. If any one level is restricted for whatever reason, the shift itself takes on the sensation of instability, and deep emotions of fear may arise. White Lightnin' aids in stabilizing the movement among these four p.e.m.s. levels when their movement is out of rhythm or out of balance. It stabilizes the multileveled synchronizing of movement within each individual and enhances the body/soul fusion, thus enabling the inner timing of change and movement to once again be reflected fully on all p.e.m.s. levels.

ROYAL HIGHNESS: (pastel pink) Final stabilization. Royal Highness relates to the full stabilization one must experience when an evolutionary step or movement has been completed. In gross terms, one might say that this is the mop-up essence. Once a conscious process has been completed, the individual has moved all aspects and levels of himself into a position of new perspective, new balance, and new awareness. There follows a period of adjustment during which the individual is completing the integration process and becoming acquainted with the results of the shift. Royal Highness helps insulate, protect, and stabilize the individual and the shift during this period when both are vulnerable.

I don't pretend to understand everything about these definitions. Sometimes when I test a need for one, and I look at how I feel along with what I'm involved in or what's going on around me at the time, the essence easily makes sense. At other times, I match what I am experiencing with the essence involved, looking at the definition, and I'll say, "Oh, so this is what that means." Or, looking at what I am experiencing along with the effects of the essence will give me a new, broader understanding of a definition I thought I had pretty well understood.

A rather graphic example of this occurred with Tomato Essence. I thought I understood the meaning of the word "shattering" as used in the definition. When I did the original translation, that word had an especially strong energy. Not long after Tomato Essence was produced, I was raising a one-week-old squirrel. He developed an intestinal block which I was unable to treat in the usual time-honored fashion — enema. He was just too tiny for even a small eyedropper. I tested him for flower essences and he tested positive for Tomato. Two hours after administration of the drops, he began to function. The block was breaking up. *That's shattering!* The rest is history and he is now grown and back in the wild. Later, I did an essence test for someone complaining of chronic constipation and, again, Tomato tested positive. She told me later that before she got home, her problem began to clear up. Since then, Tomato has tested many times over for problems in this general area. In short, I have a whole new understanding and appreciation for the word "shattering."

Then there are those times when I'll test positive for an essence, look at the definition, and have absolutely no idea why I need this one. After many years of working with the flower essences, I can only encourage you to go ahead and use it for the prescribed number of days, keeping in mind what the definition is and paying attention to how you feel. Eventually, the mystery will clear up for you, and you'll experience a whole new understanding of the definition and how it applies to you. Often, the process of clearing up the mystery is exactly what is needed in order to move beyond a situation and restore balance.

SHORT DEFINITIONS:
PERELANDRA ROSE AND GARDEN ESSENCES

In order to make these definitions easier to work with, I condensed them and now use the shortened version for quick reference when I am working with the essences. In case you'd like the convenience of the quick reference as you think about the essences, I include them here.

Perelandra Garden Essences

BROCCOLI: For the power balance that must be maintained when one perceives himself to be under siege from outside influences. Stabilizes the body/soul unit so the person won't close down, detach, and scatter.

CAULIFLOWER: Stabilizes and balances the child during the birth process.

CELERY: Restores balance of immune system during times when it is being stressed and during long-term viral or bacterial infections.

CHIVES: Reestablishes the power one has when the internal male/female dynamics are balanced and the person is functioning in a state of awareness within this balance.

COMFREY: Repairs higher vibrational soul damage that occurred in present or past lifetime.

CORN: Stabilization during spiritual expansion. Assists translation of experience into useful understanding and action.

CUCUMBER: Rebalancing during depression. Vital reattachment to life.

DILL: Assists individual in reclaiming power balance one has released to others. Victimization.

NASTURTIUM: Restores vital physical life energy during times of intense mental-level focus.

OKRA: Restores ability to see the positive in one's life and environment.

SALVIA: Restores emotional stability during times of extreme stress.

SNAP PEA: Rebalances adult or child after a nightmare. Assists ability to translate daily experience into positive process.

SUMMER SQUASH: Restores courage to the person who experiences fear and resistance when faced with daily routine. Shyness. Phobia.

SWEET BELL PEPPER: Inner peace, clarity, and calm when faced with today's stressful times. Stabilizes body/soul balance during times of stress.

TOMATO: Cleansing. Assists the body in shattering and throwing off that which is causing infection or disease.

YELLOW YARROW: Emotional protection during vulnerable times. Its support softens resistance and assists the integration process.

ZINNIA: Reconnects one to the child within. Restores playfulness, laughter, joy, and a sense of healthy priorities.

ZUCCHINI: Helps restore physical strength during convalescence.

Perelandra Rose Essences

GRUSS AN AACHEN: Stability. Balances and stabilizes the body/soul unit on all p.e.m.s. levels as it moves forward in its evolutionary process. (p.e.m.s.: physical, emotional, mental, spiritual)

PEACE: Courage. Opens the individual to the inner dynamic of courage that is aligned to universal courage.

ECLIPSE: Acceptance and insight. Enhances the individual's appreciation of his own inner knowing. Supports the mechanism that allows the body to receive the soul's input and insight.

ORANGE RUFFLES: Receptivity. Stabilizes the individual during the expansion of his sensory system.

AMBASSADOR: Pattern. Aids the individual in seeing the relationship of the part to the whole, in perceiving his pattern and purpose.

NYMPHENBURG: Strength. Supports and holds the strength created by the balance of the body/soul fusion, and facilitates the individual's ability to regain that balance.

WHITE LIGHTNIN': Synchronized movement. Stabilizes the inner timing of all p.e.m.s. levels moving in concert, and enhances the body/soul fusion.

ROYAL HIGHNESS: Final stabilization. The mop-up essence which helps to insulate, protect, and stabilize the individual and to stabilize the shift during its final stages while one is vulnerable.

GETTING YOUR OWN DEFINITIONS

You may feel inclined to produce your own flower essences. I've already given you the step-by-step production instructions. If you do, eventually you are going to be faced with a bunch of neatly labeled jars full of flower essence tincture in need of definitions. Trust me. Nothing is going to make me grouchier than getting ten requests a day from individuals who feel they need to have the essences of flowers or vegetables not listed above, and who are sure the thing I want to do most that day is get their definitions for them.

Let me give you some ideas on how to discern the definitions for yourself.

Pay attention to your intuition. If you sense that you are to make a flower essence, your intuition is already working just fine. Let it continue to carry you through the process of learning about this essence. The easy route is to sit down with pen and paper, concentrate on the essence you wish to be defined, and simply write down what comes to mind—*without* censoring it. You can check your accuracy in two ways. After using the essence for awhile, see if what you are using it for corresponds to the definition. Or, the fast, more direct check is to use kinesiology (a tool that is fully explained in the next chapter). As for a specific framework, I suggest the following.

1. Open to the Deva of Flower Essences.

Now, this is much simpler to do than you probably realize. Opening to a deva requires nothing more than a request. This may be difficult to swallow. Most people I meet who want me to help them get in contact with the devic level come prepared to roll up their sleeves, fast for six days, sweat a little blood, and arm themselves with an arsenal of crystals just in case they're really not up to the job. When I show them that all they have to do is sit down in a quiet spot, concentrate a bit on what they are doing, and just say, "I would like to be connected with the Deva of _____," they can't believe it. Then they try it, and lo and behold, they've done it and there's the deva ready to assist them.

How do they know they've connected? Simple. They use kinesiology to verify the connection. (There's that "kinesiology" word again. It's the fancy word for muscle testing. Once you read the next chapter, all the references surrounding kinesiology will fall into place for you.) Or the people proceed without this verification on the basis that truly what you ask for you receive, and devas are eager and willing to assist us humans whenever possible. This happens to be true.

The keys to getting devic information are concentration, clarity, and simplicity. Be clear about what you want and be precise about how you ask for it. As I stated before, whenever possible, state what you want aloud. Saying it audibly usually encourages us to be more precise than just thinking it.

So, to open to the Deva of Flower Essences say,
    I'd like to be connected to the Deva of Flower Essences.
Remain quiet for about ten seconds. You may feel a sensation
of energy wash over you, and then again you may feel absolutely
nothing. If you learn to use kinesiology, something I whole-
heartedly recommend, you can verify your connection by asking,
    Am I now connected to the Deva of Flower Essences?
Then test. A positive result means yes, you are connected. A
negative result means no, start over, and this time concentrate on
what you are doing. If you don't want this kind of verification, just
proceed on. When you complete the process and have an essence
definition in hand, you'll know you had help.

2. Ask (literally) the Deva of Flower Essences to give you the
balancing and healing pattern for the specific flower essence involved.

If you are getting definitions for more than one essence, be
sure to work with only one at a time. Place the jar or bottle of essence in front of you. This will clarify to the deva which essence
definition you want. When the process is completed, put that jar
to one side and place the next one in front of you. Then be sure
to ask again for the healing and balancing pattern for this essence.

3. Picture in your mind the plant and its flower. If you're having
trouble "seeing" it, look at a picture of it. (Seed catalogs are a
good source of pictures.)

This will be your starting point for the Deva of Flower Essences. It's important now that you not censor or edit your thoughts
or impressions. Release your mind to the deva. It will lead you to
a single thought or through a series of thoughts, impressions,
visuals, or sensations—whatever works best with you. Devas are

very efficient about these things and will interface with you in whatever ways you are willing to receive them and their energy. From this, you will get an idea of the balancing pattern the flower essence holds.

I'll give you an example: For cucumber, I pictured the cucumber plant and its flowers. (The picture on the front cover of this book is of cucumber flowers.) Immediately I was struck by the clear yellow color of the flowers, and the word that popped to mind was "sunshine." I stayed with that thought, and then I felt the sensation of a sunny disposition, which immediately led to a sensation of the opposite — depression. This gave me the direction of the definition, and I was off and running with the more precise and complex translation which you have read.

4. Once you get a sense of direction, ask the deva if what you are perceiving is correct.

Verbalize your perception so that you and the deva will know precisely what you think you perceived. Writing it down would be even better. If you are not disciplined in translation, for cucumber you may simply write down the word "depression" and perhaps a few words describing the sensation of depression you felt.

You can verify your perception by sensing whether or not it feels right — the old gut-instinct test. If it's not right and you remain concentrated on what you are doing (you haven't let your mind wander onto something else), you'll feel it. Something just won't feel right. The deva will be giving you the input in every possible way that will indicate the need to do it again. Go back to picturing the plant and let the deva lead you through the process again. See if the new information feels right.

If you are inclined to repeat the process just to see if you get the same results, watch out. You run a greater risk of your intellect taking over and dominating the process the second, third, and fourth times around. I suggest you stick with your first sensations and use the essence in light of this definition; then see if it holds up by corresponding with your experience.

The easiest, more efficient way I know to verify a definition, however, is through the use of kinesiology. In this process, you articulate your impressions to the Deva of Flower Essences and then ask if your impressions are correct. The deva then gives you an emphatic "yes" or "no." That answer is translated to you through the use of muscle testing, exactly as it was done in Step 1. If you test positive, it's a "yes" and the definition or perception is correct. If you test negative, it's a "no" and you need to do the process over again. The deva will work with you, giving you the experience of the healing pattern in every possible way until you are able to perceive it. So if you have to do it over, just be patient with yourself and keep at it until your perception tests positive.

5. When you have completed your work with the Deva of Flower Essences, close down the connection. Again, this is a matter of clear action—and courtesy. It lets the deva know that you wish to close for now, and it allows that disconnection to be made cleanly and efficiently. I strongly suggest that you do not remain connected indefinitely. I have found that some people think the idea of a constant devic connection sounds pretty desirable. It's not. In fact, it's an energy drain on you. Eventually you'll feel it. It's not that devas are sitting around siphoning off your energy. They don't do such things. The open connection itself is the thing that is draining energy. When you opened the connection, you orchestrated a reality (the connection between you and the deva) that requires energy in order to be maintained. To disperse that

reality, you as the orchestrator must take the responsibility of closing it down or, in other words, dismantling it.

If you forget to close down the session and remember it later or feel an energy drain that serves to remind you, just go to a quiet spot, concentrate on what you are doing, and ask that the open connection between you and the Deva of Flower Essences (or any deva you might have been working with) now be closed. You may feel a difference right away or it may take a half-hour or so for you to feel your energy level returning.

A note about the above definition process. It probably looks as if I have you going through quite an elaborate dance. Well, I do, and it's for a purpose. It's not because devas are stupid and we have to act and talk like idiots in order for them to understand us and what we want. The fact is, devas personify intelligence beyond any words I could possibly use to describe it or them. The most common breakdown (aside from disbelief) in establishing communication with the devic level or nature spirit level, or any higher level for that matter, is a lack of clarity on our part. I refer to our inability to think, write, or talk in precise, simple sentences and our equal inability to visually focus on one thing sitting before us among many things and not to stray our vision to look at the other things. When we verbally garble or slide our intent and focus around like this, the devas simply can't get a fix on what it is we want. They will not participate in our unclarity. Instead, they will wait quietly (and extremely patiently) until we are able to express ourselves precisely, simply, and clearly. They will answer our questions and address our needs in kind. In order to assist folks around these pitfalls, I set up procedures in as clear, simple, and precise a manner as possible, and I utilize as much clarifying action as possible. Hence, the dance.

If you wish to know more about how to work with the devas and nature spirits in general, I again recommend the *Perelandra Garden Workbook.*

PERELANDRA ROSE ESSENCES II: A NEW SET

This set of Perelandra flower essences developed in 1992. The eight essences are made from roses growing in the Perelandra garden and address the specific balancing and stabilizing needs of the body's central nervous system. They also address the functions within the central nervous system that are activated and/or impacted during a *deep expansion experience.* Here, one is not simply processing ordinary, everyday occurrences. Rather, one is faced with an experience that is new and challenging to the present balance and functioning of the body. When faced with this kind of expansion, the central nervous system is required to function in new ways, and with patterns and rhythms yet to be experienced. The Rose Essences II address this phenomenon by balancing and stabilizing this system's functions that have been impacted by the expansion.

I wish I could list specific experiences that would identify deep expansion situations for you, but a deep expansion for some is an everyday life process for others. The only thing I can say is that if you are interested in Perelandra processes and incorporating flower essences in your life, you are the kind of person who doesn't shy away from deep expansion. I think it would be good to have this set handy.

The following are the short definitions for Rose II. The name of each essence is the same as the rose from which it is made.

BLAZE IMPROVED CLIMBING ROSE: Softens and relaxes first the central nervous system and then the body as a whole, thus allowing the input from an expansion experience to be appropriately sorted, shifted and integrated within the body.

MAYBELLE STEARNS: Stabilizes and supports the sacrum during an expansion experience.

MR. LINCOLN: Balances and stabilizes the cerebrospinal fluid (CSF) pulse while it alters its rhythm and patterning to accommodate the expansion.

SONIA: Stabilizes and supports the CSF pulse *after* it has completed its shift to accommodate the expansion.

CHICAGO PEACE: Stabilizes movement of and interaction among the cranial bones, CSF and sacrum during an expansion experience.

BETTY PRIOR: Stabilizes and balances the delicate rhythm of expansion and contraction of the cranial bones during the expansion.

TIFFANY: Stabilizes the cranials as they shift their alignment appropriately to accommodate the input and impulses of expansion.

OREGOLD: Stabilizes and balances the cranials, central nervous system, CSF and sacrum after an expansion process is complete.

ADDITIONAL ESSENCES DEVELOPMENTS

The Perelandra Nature Program Essences were developed in 1993, and Perelandra Soul Ray Essences were developed in 1994. For full descriptions of these two extraordinary essence sets, please see the Perelandra catalog. The Nature Program and Soul Ray Essences sets combined with the Rose, Garden and Rose II Sets cover a full range of an individual's essence needs.

4

Kinesiology:
the Tool for Testing

WHEN IT COMES TO FINDING OUT which flower essence you need, I suggest you use kinesiology—muscle testing. Now, I know it's easier to look at each of the bottles and select the one(s) that intuitively attract your attention. That works. And if it feels more comfortable to you, by all means do it. Also, you can read the list of definitions and intellectually discern which essences you need in light of how you are feeling and what's happening around you.

But one thing I've learned time and time again throughout my years of using the essences is that sometimes our inner state can be more complex than we realize, and perceiving accurate needs can be tricky. And often, we can be going through a situation that we are absolutely sure, just on the intensity level alone, has to be throwing us out of kilter and overloading or disconnecting every electrical circuit we have. Or something seemingly commonplace and insignificant has occurred and we would bet the mortgage we're breezing through this thing with terrific ease and grace. Then we test, using kinesiology, and find out we're wrong all the way around. Just because something is intense doesn't mean we've fallen apart. On the contrary, we seem to know how to hold up under a lot of adversity. And the opposite can be true about what looks to be the little stuff when, in fact, the little stuff often carries with it a lot of subtle nuances that can broadside us.

The best way through the forest that I know of is to use kinesiology. It allows us to discern what we need and don't need, despite what we think. And by getting that kind of accurate feedback, we learn more about ourselves. We learn about our strength when we test for essences during a time of total disaster and find out we're doing okay. It also reveals to us our patterns of how we over-respond to other situations. Again we learn. If we wish to change the pattern, we now have an idea of how it affects and weakens us, and when.

Kinesiology is simple. Everybody is set up for it because it links you to your electrical system and your muscles. If you are alive, you have these two things. I know that sounds smart-mouthed of me, but I've learned that sometimes people refuse to believe something can be so simple. So they create a mental block on the basis that only "sensitive types" can do this, or only women can do this. It's just not true. Kinesiology just happens to be one of those simple things in life that's waiting around to be learned and used by everyone.

If you've ever been to a chiropractor or wholistic physician, chances are you've experienced kinesiology. The doctor tells you to stick out your arm and resist his pressure. It feels like he's trying to push your arm down, and he's told you not to let him do it. Everything is going fine, and then all of a sudden he presses and your arm falls down like a floppy fish. That's kinesiology.

Let me explain: If a negative energy (that is, any physical object or energy that does not maintain or enhance the health and balance of an individual) is introduced into a person's overall energy field, either within the body or in the immediate environment outside the body, his muscles, when having physical pressure applied, will be unable to hold their power. In other words, if pressure is applied to an individual's extended arm while his field is being affected by a negative, the arm will not be able to resist the pressure. It will weaken and fall to his side. In the case of the physician or chiropractor, they are testing specific areas of the body. When making contact with a weakened area, the muscles respond by losing their power. If pressure is applied while connecting with a positive or balanced area, the person will easily be able to resist and the arm will hold its position.

To expand further, when a negative is placed within a person's field, his electrical system (that electrical grid we've been talking about that is contained within and surrounds the body) will immediately respond by "short-circuiting," making it difficult for the muscles to maintain their strength and hold the position when pressure is added. When a positive is placed within the field, the electrical system holds and the muscles are able to maintain their level of strength when pressure is applied.

This electrical/muscular relationship is a natural part of the human system. It is not mystical or magical. Kinesiology is the established method for reading their state of interaction at any given moment.

If you have ever experienced muscle testing, you most likely participated in the above-described, two-man operation. You provided the extended arm and the other person provided the pressure. Although efficient, this can sometimes be cumbersome when you want to test something on your own. Arm pumpers have the nasty habit of disappearing right when you need them the most. So you'll be learning to self-test — no arm pumpers needed.

KINESIOLOGY SELF-TESTING STEPS

1. THE CIRCUIT FINGERS: **If you are right-handed:** Place your left hand palm up. Connect the tip of your left thumb with the tip of the left little finger (*not your index finger*). **If you are left-handed:** Place your right hand palm up. Connect the tip of your right thumb with the tip of your right little finger. By connecting your thumb and little finger, you have just closed an electrical circuit in your hand, and it is this circuit you will use for testing.

Before going on, look at the position you have just formed with

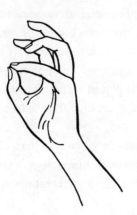

your hand. If your thumb is touching the tip of your index or first finger, laugh at yourself for not being able to follow directions and change the position to touch the tip of the thumb with the tip of the little or fourth finger. Most likely this will not feel at all comfortable to you. If you are feeling a weird sense of awkwardness, you've got the first step of the test position! In time, the hand and fingers will adjust to being put in this position and it will feel fine.

2. THE TEST FINGERS: To test the circuit (the means by which you will apply pressure to yourself), place the thumb and index finger of your other hand inside the circle you have created by connecting your thumb and little finger. The thumb/index finger should be right under the thumb/little finger, touching them. Don't try to make a circle with your test fingers. They're just placed inside the circuit fingers which do form a circle. It will look as if the circuit fingers are resting on the test fingers.

3. Keeping this position, ask yourself a yes/no question in which you already know the answer to be yes. ("Is my name ____?") Once you've asked the question, press your circuit fingers together, keeping the tip-to-tip position. *Using the same amount of pressure,* try to pull apart the circuit fingers with your test fingers. Press the lower thumb against the upper thumb, the lower index finger against the upper little finger.

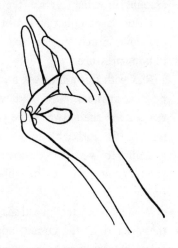

Another way to say all of this is that the circuit position described in Step 1 replaces the position you take when you stick your arm out for the physician. The testing position in Step 2 is in place of the physician or other convenient arm pumper. After you ask the yes/no question and you press your circuit fingers tip-to-tip, that's equal to the doctor saying, "Resist my pressure." Your circuit fingers have now become your outstretched, stiffened arm. Trying to pull apart those fingers with your testing fingers is equal to the doctor pressing down on your arm.

If the answer to the question is positive (if your name is what you think it is!), you will not be able to easily pull apart the circuit fingers. The electrical circuit will hold, your muscles will maintain their strength, and your circuit fingers will not separate. You will feel the strength in that circuit. *Important:* Be sure the amount of pressure holding together the circuit fingers is equal to the amount pressing against them with your testing fingers. Also, don't use a pumping action in your testing fingers when trying to pry your circuit fingers apart. Use an equal, steady, and continuous pressure.

Play with this a bit. Ask a few more yes/no questions that have positive answers. Now, I know it's going to seem that if you already know the answer to be yes, you are probably "throwing" the test. That's reasonable to feel, but for the time being, until you get a feeling for what the positive response feels like in your fingers, you're going to need to deliberately ask yourself questions with positive answers.

While asking the questions, if you are having trouble sensing the strength of the circuit, apply a little more pressure. Or consider that you may be applying too much pressure and pull back

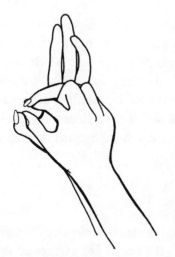

some. You don't have to break or strain your fingers for this; you just have to add enough pressure to make them feel alive, connected, and alert.

4. Once you have a clear sense of the positive response, ask yourself a question that has a negative answer. Again press your circuit fingers together and, using equal pressure, press against the circuit fingers with the test fingers. This time the electrical circuit will break and the circuit fingers will weaken and separate. Because the electrical circuit is broken, the muscles in the circuit fingers don't have the power to hold the fingers together. In a positive state, the electrical circuit holds and the muscles have the power to keep the two fingers together.

Play with negative questions a bit, and then return to positive questions. Get a good feeling for the strength between your circuit fingers when the electricity is in a positive state and the weakness when the electricity is in a negative state. You can even ask yourself (your own system) for a positive response and then, after testing, ask for a negative response. ("Give me a positive response." Test. "Give me a negative response." Test.) You will feel the positive strength and the negative weakness. In the beginning, you may feel only a slight difference between the two. With practice, that difference will become more pronounced. For now, it's just a matter of trusting what you've learned — and practice.

Don't forget the overall concept behind kinesiology. What enhances our body, mind, and soul makes us strong. Together, our body, mind, and soul create a wholistic environment which, when balanced, is strong and solid. If something enters into that environment that negates or challenges the balance, the entire environment is weakened. The state of that strength or weakness is registered in the electrical system, and through muscle testing it can be discerned.

Kinesiology Tips

If you are having trouble feeling the electrical circuit on the circuit fingers, try switching hands—the circuit fingers become the testing fingers and vice versa. Most people who are right-handed have this particular electrical circuitry in their left hand. Left-handers generally have the circuitry in their right hand. But sometimes a right-hander has the circuitry in the right hand and a left-hander has it in the left hand. You may be one of those people.

If you have an injury such as a muscle sprain in either hand or arm, don't try to learn kinesiology until you have healed. Kinesiology is muscle testing, and a muscle injury will interfere with the testing—and the testing will interfere with the healing of the muscle injury.

Also, while first learning kinesiology, do yourself a favor and set aside some quiet time to go through the instructions and play with the testing. Trying to learn this while riding the New York subway during evening rush hour isn't going to give you the break you need. Once you have learned, you'll be able to test all kinds of things while riding the subway.

Sometimes I meet people who are trying to learn kinesiology and aren't having much luck. They've gotten frustrated, decided this isn't for them, and gone on to try to learn another means of testing. Well, I'll listen to them explaining what they did, and before they know it, I've verbally tricked them with a couple of suggestions about their testing, which they'll try, and they're feeling kinesiology for the first time – a strong 'yes' and a clear 'no.' The problem wasn't kinesiology. Everyone, as I have said, has an electrical system. The problem was that they wanted to learn it so much that they became overly anxious and tense – they blocked.

So, since you won't have me around to trick you, I suggest that if you suspect you're blocking, go ahead on to something else. Then trick yourself. When you care the least about whether or not you learn kinesiology, start playing with it again. Approach it as if it were a game. *Then* you'll feel the strength and weakness in the fingers.

Now, suppose the testing has been working fine, and then suddenly you can't get a clear result (what I call a "definite maybe") or get no result at all. Check:

1. Sloppy testing. You try to press apart the fingers before applying pressure between the circuit fingers. This happens especially when we've been testing for awhile and become over-confident or very quick in the testing process. I think it happens to all of us from time to time and serves to remind us to keep our attention on the matter at hand. (Excuse the lousy pun.)

2. External distractions. Trying to test in a noisy or active area can cause you to lose your concentration. The testing will feel unsure or contradict itself if you double-check by testing the results

again. Often, simply moving to a quiet, calm spot and concentrating on what you are doing will be just what's needed for successful testing.

3. Focus/concentration. Even in a quiet spot, one's mind may wander and the testing will feel fuzzy, weak, or contradictory. It's important to retain concentration throughout the process. Check how you are feeling. If you're tired, I suggest you not try to test until you've rested a bit. And if you have to go to the bathroom, do it. That little situation is a sure concentration-destroyer.

4. The question isn't clear. A key to kinesiology is asking a *simple* yes/no question, not two questions in one, each having a possible yes/no answer. When testing for flower essences, make sure you are asking one question at a time.

5. You must want to accept the results of the test. If you enter a kinesiology test not wanting to "hear" the answer, for whatever reason, you can override the test with your emotions and your will. This is true for conventional situations as well. If you really don't want something to work for you, it won't work. That's our personal power dictating the outcome.

Also, if you are trying to do testing during a situation that is especially emotional for you, that deeply stirs your emotions, or if you are trying to ask a question in which you have a strong, personal investment in the answer—such as, "Should I buy this beautiful $250,000 house?"—I suggest that you not do any testing until you are calmer or can get some emotional distance from the situation. During such times, you're walking a very fine line between a clear test and a test that your desires are overriding. Kinesiology as a tool isn't the question here. It's the condition or intent of the tester that's at issue. In fact, some questions just shouldn't be asked, but *which* questions are relative to who's doing the asking. We each need to develop discernment around which questions are appropriate for us to ask.

If you are in an emergency situation, for example, and have no choice but to test someone close who might need flower essences, be aware of your emotional vulnerability. When I am involved with testing during emotionally stressful times, I will stop for a moment, collect my thoughts, and make a personal commitment to concentrate on the testing only. If I need to test an emotionally charged question or a question about something I have a personal investment in, I will stop a moment, commit myself to the test, and open myself to receiving *the* answer and not the answer I might desire.

QUESTIONS AND THE UNIVERSE

You might have guessed by now that kinesiology is a tool that can be used for getting answers about things besides whether or not we need a flower essence. In fact, it is a wonderful tool for getting all kinds of information. More than once I've had the experience, when teaching kinesiology, of someone in the group bursting into tears when they suddenly realized that because of what they have just learned, they have access to the answer to any question they have ever asked. I would feel irresponsible if I didn't discuss these other opportunities with kinesiology and the care with which one should use them. It would be as if I'd given you a powerful tool and only half the instructions. So what follows is more information on kinesiology and the issues surrounding it, beyond what you will need for testing the flower essences.

I've already stated that one of the keys to kinesiology is asking a simple question in a yes/no format. I can go even further with this and say that one of the keys to receiving *any* information or insight from intelligent sources beyond our conscious selves is the ability to ask a clear, concise question regarding the information we'd like to know. I can also say that the biggest stumbling block to the interlevel information flow, besides the fear that we can't "hear," has to do with asking questions.

Over the years, I've learned some mighty lessons in this area. I've found out that there exists in the universe what I call a "cosmic code of conduct." Our worth as free-thinking individuals is recognized and deferred to by all other intelligences. The universe isn't going to throw truckloads of information at us at will. We must indicate that we wish to know these things. And we must indicate precisely what areas of knowledge we are referring to. It is not enough for me to say I want to know everything there is to know. In order to receive a response to my desire to know, I must express what precisely it is I wish to know. The universe looks to me to take responsibility for the timing of my growth and expansion. Indicating what I'm ready to learn through the tool of asking a question is how I express my timing to all outside me.

In *Behaving . . .*, I talk about what it meant for me to accept my position as creator of the garden. This required that I establish my rightful position as co-creator with the nature intelligences. It also required that I recognize my responsibility to do this. To be in any lesser position would place me on a level of the ignorant servant. This is unacceptable to the intelligences I work with and, as far as I am aware, it is unacceptable to the universe at large. By accepting our responsibility to make known what we wish to learn for the purpose of expansion and growth, we accept our position as creator of our personal garden.

One consideration within the cosmic code of conduct has to do with timing—specifically, the universal acknowledgment of our personal timing. This is why we don't get truckloads of information coming at us from out of the blue. The following is an excerpt from a monograph called "Timing," which I received in 1984 from Universal Light.

UNIVERSAL LIGHT

The process of evolution is continuous within each soul. And by association, so is the concept of timing, since it is so intimately linked to evolution. Therefore, if a man can point to only a handful of moments in which timing played a role, he has missed observing and very likely experiencing the many instances of timing in his life. If one were to see his life as a tapestry of design and color, the pattern of the weave comes significantly from timing. As man recognizes and responds to the phenomenon of timing, the weave in his tapestry becomes more dramatic and the color more brilliant. It is his choice. There are a number of phenomena available to him which he can choose to incorporate—at any level of intensity he desires—into his life.

Nothing in the universe, in all of reality, is held back from the individual living on Earth. Each person decides for himself the intensity with which he chooses to live his life. The limitations are his own. How much is available to him is not dictated by the universe. It is entirely dictated by the individual. Most souls who live on Earth, as they struggle through their lessons concerning the

relationship of spirit flowing through form, feel that the universe
and its truths are being held back from them in one degree or
another because they are encased — or enslaved — in the body. This
is not only untrue, it is an excuse. To think that something greater
than yourself is dictating what you should or should not know,
deprives you of the responsibility for self-growth, self-evolution.
What is the use of working and seeking to improve, to open and ex-
pand yourself when you think you are dictated to by some intel-
ligence, some consciousness greater than yourself, outside of your-
self.

The evolutionary process in all souls involves the shifting and ex-
panding of an individual's boundaries and limitations, or what has
been termed the "ring-pass-not." [Ring-pass-not: The boundary or
scope of limitations we each have that separates our working and
workable knowledge and reality from the rest of all knowledge
and reality.] *Do not think that when we use the word "limitation"*
we are being judgmental. All souls have some aspect of limitation.
There is wise limitation and there is limitation that derives from
fear. Wise limitation defines the individual who knows what level
and part of reality he can enfold into his life and successfully in-
tegrate into his actions in form. Wise limitation admits that
knowledge and reality which can be fully grounded by an individual.
A wise man understands what he can take into his conscious know-
ing and what he can ground in action during his life. It is a sign of
wisdom when he can say "enough," and give himself time to in-
tegrate that which he has come to understand, to successfully reflect
it through his body, his actions, and into form. Once successfully
grounded, he can shift his ring-pass-not and take in more.

I've had another major lesson around this issue of questions, and that has to do with the difference between asking a question of the intellect and asking a question that gives me information for integration. These are fairly easy things to distinguish between on paper but a bit tough to begin to discern personally.

You see, we live in an age where we are given deference and approval for the amount of information we know. Our school system honors the student who can stuff a lot of information in his head and then repeat it at the correct moment. Not only do we admire individuals who can do this, but we grow up believing that to live well in society, one must remain intellectually alert. Ask questions. Take in information.

I don't mean to imply that there is something wrong with our being intellectually alert and developed. But I do point out the pitfall that has encouraged us to develop the habit of asking questions for the sake of asking questions. We do nothing more with the answer than file it. This is what I mean by an intellectual question. The more I have developed around this issue of asking questions, the more I have realized what a useless exercise it is for me to ask an intellectual question. What in the world can I do with all that information?

The integration question is one in which the answer is received in right timing, and we are able to integrate the information we receive into our life. It can change the way we think, how we perceive the reality around us, how we act, and how we move through our daily schedule. When this type of question is asked, we are able to move the answer through a complete experiential grounding process.

I can't give you a formula for distinguishing an intellectual question from an integration question. Obviously, since we are all different, what is intellectual for one is integration for another. But I can give you some hints I've come up with in my own journey through the question issue.

One of the best ways to begin weeding out needless information-gathering is to start making it a practice to act on every piece of information we take in. Just the thought of this will give us mental strain. Very quickly, as we attempt to respond, time itself will encourage us to be more discerning about the information we are gathering. There simply isn't enough time in the day to respond with some form of action to all the pieces of information we take in. We would die of exhaustion.

I experienced a gradual change about asking questions. At first I continued to ask all the questions that typically popped into mind. As I began to understand the wisdom of taking in only the information I could integrate and use, I became sensitive to what was happening when I asked a question. I could feel some answers move as an energy right into my body system. Other answers I felt bounce off me as a rubber ball off a brick wall. I could physically hear what was being said to me, but the energy behind what was being said didn't come into me. I wasn't comprehending or retaining what was being said. After awhile, I could anticipate the effect an answer would have on me—I could feel whether the energy was going to absorb into me or bounce off— and know that I need not bother to go through the exercise of physically hearing it. I'd just apologize for asking the question and indicate that I need not hear the answer. Further down the line, I realized I could think the question, feel the impact of the answer on me, and make a decision whether or not to even open my mouth.

So, here you sit with kinesiology, something that can give you easy access to any information that exists. It can open that door to you. And that's precisely what I want to happen for you. But I want to encourage you to use kinesiology as a viable living tool within your daily life, not as a tool to become cosmic scholars. I want you to use it to participate more fully in your life and your environment. I don't want to encourage armchair observers. You can easily bog yourself down with information overload and render yourself motionless. Or frantically run around in a hundred directions at once trying to do something about everything, and end up accomplishing nothing.

THE NUTS AND BOLTS OF ASKING A QUESTION

Remember that to use kinesiology successfully, you have to rely on questions in a yes/no format. Short, simple, concise questions. This is easy—and it's not so easy! As thinking adults, we have learned to use compound and compound-complex question frameworks. After all, we don't want to sound like idiots. Simple questions are out of style, and consequently we are out of practice. However, with a little bit of thought put to the issue, we can learn to rephrase any question we might have or anything we wish to know into a yes/no format.

I'll give you some common pitfalls to watch out for.

Let's say you want to know if the beautifully blooming yellow marigolds in your backyard flower garden should be made into a flower essence. You open to the Deva of Flower Essences (using the same process as described in the flower essence-making process) and ask, "Should I make an essence from the flowers of the yellow marigolds in my garden?" Not, "Gee, those marigolds look so pretty and I bet they would make a nice essence but then maybe I shouldn't pick them and disturb the plants but I just know that something that beautiful is powerful and surely the plants wouldn't mind if I picked a couple of flowers but then maybe its too late in the season to make a good essence . . ." The first response the deva would make to you, if it could get through at all, is, "What is your question?"

I call asking a strung-out question like this "mashed potatoing." In essence, all you've presented the deva with is a shapeless glob of mashed potatoes, thus giving no clear avenue for response. If you are faced with an issue that involves many considerations, simply present each consideration separately in a yes/no format. For example, if I were to break down the mashed potato question, I would present it something like this:

Would a flower essence from the yellow marigold in my garden be beneficial to me and my family? (yes/no)

Should I make this flower essence soon? (yes/no)

Are these flowers ready for essence-making now? (yes/no)

(If not, and it's late in the season) Should I wait until next spring and make an essence from the early yellow marigold flowers? (yes/no)

Will picking the necessary flowers disturb the plants? (yes/no)

Does exceptional beauty in the flowers correlate with the amount of power of the healing pattern it holds? (yes/no)

(If you should make the essence immediately) Are there specific flowers I should use? (yes/no)

(If yes) Point to flowers individually and ask for each,
    Is it this one? (yes/no)
    This one? (yes/no)
    This one? (yes/no)
I've not only shown you how to break down a complicated situation into a series of simple yes/no questions, I've also shown how you can build your question process based on the answer to each question. This is how you receive complex information with lots of nuances – allow the answer to the previous question to guide you to ask the next question and keep the process building.

What you are doing is playing *Twenty Questions* with a deva. This may seem tedious to you, but this kind of simplicity is an excellent place to begin when learning something new. Don't let false pride and the fear of looking silly get in your way. If you take the time to build your foundation, eventually you will develop refinements to your technique.

Part of my development has centered around the use of intuition. Once I began to feel comfortable with the *Twenty Questions* routine, I noticed that my intuition began to play into it. I paid attention to this and soon realized that the nature intelligence I was connected with was using my intuition to guide me more efficiently through the questions. I got to the point where, if I was walking through the garden and I suddenly and clearly thought about flower essences, I would connect with the Deva of Flower Essences and ask:
    Am I to make a flower essence? (yes)
Then my attention would be drawn to a specific flower or I'd get an intuitive hit about a specific flower, and I would ask, in light of the new input:
    Am I to make an essence from the yellow marigolds? (yes)

As you can see, I was able to get to the heart of the matter comparatively quickly. But intuition wasn't added until I felt comfortable with the more basic technique. As with any tool, the better we are with the basics, the more proficient we'll be with what develops later. I suggest patience while you are in the beginning process of learning. Develop a sense of ease with the basic techniques, and rather than get into a competitive achievement contest with yourself, allow further refinements to develop gradually and on their own. If you have patience, this will automatically happen.

Either/Or Situations

I find myself faced with either/or situations quite frequently. This is simple to deal with. Let's say you must do something and you have two or more options as possibilities. For example: You get out of bed one morning with a driving desire to wear your yellow and green polka dot shirt. Then you saunter to the closet and, as you look for your snappy yellow and green polka dot shirt, your eye catches the purple and orange striped one, and you're overcome with an equal desire to wear this one. Being a responsible person who desires to participate in the universal flow on a daily basis, you say to yourself, "Well, which one should I wear?" The 'Well, which one is it?' question is a sure sign you are in an either/or situation. In such situations, I will ask first, "Does it matter which one of these two shirts I wear today?" (If I get a no, I can exercise free will and make a personal decision based on which shirt attracts me the most. If I get a yes, then I'll shift into a yes/no format and list each shirt separately to find out which one it's to be.)

In the above scenario, I imply a connection to my own higher self by asking myself direct questions. We have housed, on the level of the higher self, all the information about ourselves. In situations where the information requested has a more serious impact on us and our lives, we may wish not just to imply this connection but to consciously make it, very much as we would consciously connect with the Deva of Flower Essences before beginning to ask flower essence questions. To connect with my higher self, all I do is direct my attention into my higher self for about five seconds. If this seems nebulous to you, just say aloud:

I wish to be connected to my own higher self.

Focus your attention on what you are saying. Or think up a simple, visual symbol you can use for your higher self. It can be anything that symbolizes something special about your higher self. I once had a woman use a fresh-baked apple pie as her symbol. I have no idea what the connection was for her, but it worked like a charm every time she wanted a conscious connection. After saying, "I wish to be connected to my own higher self," spend five or ten seconds thinking of your symbol. If you want confirmation, test yourself using kinesiology.

Am I now connected to my own higher self? (yes)

Am I clear to ask questions? (yes)

Which of these two shirts should I wear?

The one with yellow and green polka dots? (no)

The one with purple and orange stripes? (Yes, but I still think you could upgrade your sense of fashion!)

A Note on Clarity

If you're having difficulty wording a simple yes/no question, consider this an important issue to be faced and something worth spending the time to rectify. You have not simply stumbled upon a glitch in your quest to use kinesiology. You've also stumbled upon a glitch in the communication between your higher self and your conscious self. If you can't even clearly word the question, you can't expect an answer. I have met people who cannot articulate a question. In a workshop they will attempt to ask me something and I can't figure out what they are asking — nor can anyone else in the workshop. Usually it turns out that they are frustrated because they can't get any clarity in their own life and are trying to ask me what to do about it.

For those of you who find yourselves in this boat, you have a terrific opportunity to turn that around and develop internal order by putting effort into learning how to articulate a simple yes/no question. In this instance, you are not only developing the tool of kinesiology, you are also developing the clarity for communicating with yourself. I fully understand that it will take focus on your part, and in comparison to someone who finds articulating a simple question easy, to you it will seem herculean. But if you wish to function consciously with your many levels, you must provide internal clarity and order.

I recommend that you initially devote your attention to learning to ask simple questions and not worry about receiving answers. When you need to ask someone a question, take time to consider what you really want to ask and how it can be most clearly and efficiently worded. It helps to write down the question. In this way, you can visually see your words. If they don't convey what you mentally want to express, play with the wording. Keep doing this until you feel those words accurately and concisely communicate what you wish to ask. Then go to that person and ask the question. Notice the difference in quality of how the person answers you. Your clarity will inspire similar clarity in the response.

I urge you to continue this process for a fair period of time — even dedicating yourself to the process for awhile. Quite often, that frustrating inner confusion exists because we've not had an acceptable framework for the development of mental ordering. Learning to ask questions gives the mind something tangible to work with and, in the process, you learn mind-word-and-mouth coordination. You'll find that as you develop the ability to clearly articulate a question, your inner fog will begin to lift, which in turn will automatically begin to lift your outer fog.

FINAL COMMENTS ON KINESIOLOGY

Kinesiology is like any tool. The more you practice, the better you are at using it. You'll need a sense of confidence about using this tool, especially when you are in the midst of getting some very strange answers to what you thought were pretty straight questions. It helps you to get over the initial "this-is-too-weird-and-the-damned-testing-isn't-working" stage if you have some confidence in your ability to feel a clear positive and negative response. The only way I know over this hump is to practice testing. You will develop clarity in your testing. You'll learn your personal pitfalls.

I have found in teaching kinesiology that something very interesting happens to some people when they are learning it. Every block, doubt, question, and personal challenge they have, when faced head-on with something perceived as unconventional, comes right to the surface. It's as if the physical tool of kinesiology itself serves to bring to the surface all those hurdles. So they learn kinesiology right away and are using it well, when all of a sudden it's not working for them. In their talking to me about it, I find out that the thing they are doing differently now that they didn't do at first is double-checking their answers — and rechecking, and rechecking, and doing it again, and again . . . Each time the answers vary or the fingers get mushy and they get definite maybes.

Well, again the issue isn't the kinesiology. The issue is really why they are suddenly going through all this rechecking business. The things that have surfaced for them are the questions around trust in their own ability, belief that such unconventional things really do happen and are happening to them, and a sudden outpouring of lack of self-confidence.

The only way I know over this kind of hurdle is to defy it — keep testing. The other alternative is to succumb to it and stop developing with kinesiology. That doesn't really prove anything. So in cases like this, I suggest the person keep testing, *stop double-checking*, and take the plunge to go with their first testing result. Eventually the consequences and outcome of what is done based on the first test result will in themselves verify the accuracy of the testing. From this, your confidence builds. I firmly believe that only clear personal evidence can get us through these kinds of hurdles and blocks — and that means just continuing to go on.

So, what can we practice test on? Everything. You could easily drive yourself nuts. What you should wear. What you should wear for a special event. What would be healthiest for you to eat for breakfast, lunch, and dinner. You take ten separate vitamin and mineral supplements as a matter of course on a daily basis. Try testing them individually ("Do I need vitamin E? B₆? Iron?") to see if you need all ten every day. Or if there are some you don't need to take at all. You are sitting at a restaurant and they don't have Tofu Supreme on the menu. Is there anything on that menu that is perfectly healthy for you to eat? ("Should I eat fish?" [yes/no] "Should I eat beef?" [yes/no] "Chicken?" [yes/no] "Häagen-Dazs fudge ripple ice cream?" [Yes!!]) And one thing you can frequently test yourself for is whether or not you need flower essences.

The point is to test everything you possibly can that doesn't place you in a life-threatening situation, follow through on your answers, and then look at the results. As I have worked through the years to refine my ability to use kinesiology, I have, on many occasions, purposely followed through on answers that made no sense at all to me, just to see if the testing was accurate. Doing this and looking at the results with a critical eye is the only way I know to learn about ourselves as kinesiology testers and to discover the nuances and uses of kinesiology itself.

One last piece of information: Give yourself about a year to develop confidence with kinesiology. Now, you'll be able to use it right away. This just takes sticking with your initial efforts until you get those first feelings of positive strength and negative weakness in the circuit fingers. But I have found from my own experience and from watching others that it takes about a year of experimentation, to fully learn the art of asking accurate yes/no questions, and to tackle the hurdles. As one woman said this summer, "You stick with this stuff a year, and boy, what a great thing you end up with!"

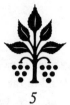

5

When to Use Flower Essences

SOMETIMES IT IS VERY EASY to know if you need flower essences. You're sitting in a chair, eyes watering, nose running, sneezing, coughing, achey all over—in general, you look like one of those cold-remedy ads on television. Take a hint and test yourself for the essences. In fact, any time you are sick or feel something "coming on," you can take that as a sign to test for flower essences.

Remember that by the time you are sick, you are using the flower essences not as a preventative but as part of what you need to do in order to get healthy again. You already know you have electrical circuitry that has overloaded or broken. The fact that you are sick is telling you this. The road back to health is greatly enhanced if you use the essences and allow them to do their job of reconnecting and stabilizing the weakened electrical areas while the body goes through the necessary healing process.

Also, if you're sick, your body is telling you that something in your life is affecting you to the point where it is no longer possible to maintain healthy physical balance. By testing the essences (a process I will describe in detail in the next chapter), you are able to identify precisely which essence you need in order to reestablish electrical balance. At the same time, the definition of that essence gives you an idea of what in your life is causing the problem.

Now, one thing I feel is important to watch out for when using the flower essences is the inclination to become judgmental. People either become embarrassed over the fact that they might test for a need for essences and translate this as meaning that there is something wrong with their character, or they get into an inferior/superior kind of judgment based on who around them needs essences, and who is more perfect and doesn't need them. They make it into a contest, the loser being the one who needs the most essences. The whole thing is nuts and just points out how little is understood about flower essences and about what is happening to someone when they become ill.

I like to think of each of us holding a circle about eight inches in diameter. From a point at the very center of that circle radiate countless numbers of hairlike lines that stretch all the way to the outer edge of the circle. Each line represents an emotion or trait. We all have a circle full of the same emotions and traits. It's standard equipment that gets activated at birth. To me, balance means all of those lines are active and operating *within* the boundary of the circle. Life experiences impact the circle, causing appropriate action and interaction of the lines. When we maintain our balance during any specific experience, it just means the lines are still contained within the circle. However, some experiences can impact us, and one or more lines suddenly shoot out beyond the perimeter of the circle. The experiences, for whatever reason, are either new, unusual, and out of the norm, or come with an especially difficult twist to them. We don't just react, we over-react. And it's the overreaction that causes the complementary lines, those lines related to the overreaction, to shoot out beyond the circle's perimeters. This causes the electrical circuitry to over-load or break.

To continue the imagery of the circle, taking a flower essence does not eliminate the shooting line. By balancing or reconnecting the circuitry, it returns the stretch of the line to *within* the perimeter of the circle. So, let's say you and I have a very close friend in common, and that friend, for whatever reason, decides to instantly and completely cut all ties with both of us and begins to spread really vicious but untrue stories about us. Well, it would be appropriate for you and me to feel shock, pain, anger, hurt, even grief and depression. We both test to see if we need essen-ces and find that you need nothing and I need Cucumber Es-sence. This means I'm so depressed by this that my "depression" line is shooting way out of my circle. It does not mean that you are not depressed by this. Instead, you are *appropriately* depressed. To take it further, it doesn't even say I am feeling a greater intensity of depression than you. All my need for Cucum-ber Essence is saying is that this particular situation is causing me to overreact in the area of depression, and that overreaction is relative to my personal framework of balance, not yours. If we could take my overreaction and superimpose it onto you, we might still find that you do not need Cucumber Essence. You're still doing fine.

Yet we could take a similar scenario and have another mutual friend do approximately the same thing to us (You and I need a new group of friends!), and this time around *you* may need the

Cucumber Essence or another related essence and I need nothing. This means that this particular time, for whatever reason, your "depression" line shot out and mine stayed within the circle. It still says nothing about which one of us has more feeling in these situations. It only tells us which one just blew a circuit.

In all of this, there's absolutely nothing to judge. Nobody is "better" for not needing flower essences and nobody is lesser for needing them — just smart for using them.

In my role as a flower essences practitioner and teacher, I've also had to deal with the notion that others hold that at some magical point, if we keep trudging forward, it all comes together for us (whatever that means) and we suddenly function perfectly. First of all, to maintain that notion requires one to believe that anything less than perfection (the definition of perfection changes from person to person) is a problem, or wrong, or "below." In terms of health and illness, this becomes a very difficult dynamic with which to work. A person with this notion sees illness as failure or as a sign that one is beneath perfection. It plays right into their feelings of self-worth and quite often translates into a subconscious belief that they are not worthy of good health. I see my health as a sign to me that right now, as of this present moment, whoever I am and whatever I am dealing with are in a state of balance. If tomorrow I should get sick, or feel fine but test that I need an essence, I read that as a sign of change and a need to discover new balance in light of new input and information. Everything I've learned and all the changes I've made up to that point cannot be looked at suddenly as being wrong, and I didn't fail at getting myself through life just because at this particular point I'm sick or out of balance. In other words, I wasn't sitting on that great point of perfection yesterday and then suddenly, because of some failure on my part, tumble off of it today.

Another thought. From everything I've learned, both from working in the garden with the nature intelligences and from the various other sources I've been lucky to work with, everything, including us, is constantly and forever evolving. I've learned that being alive is another way of expressing one's participation in this continuous forward motion. It is my experience that as soon as I think I'm "getting myself together," as soon as I get that nice, comfortable feeling of complacency, that thing inside me that keeps me connected with life starts sending out those goofy signals again, and there I am feeling the need for forward motion. Complacency just flew out the window, and I'm now busy reordering the necessary parts of my life in order to create a new balance. Quite frankly, I don't think there is one, single point of perfection out there. Every time we begin to feel near it, the ante goes up, we expand in some new way, and we have to develop a different framework and tools for living this new life well. Evolution — it never stops.

So how does all of this fit into flower essences and health? If one sees life as a series of forward-moving changes rather than a single point of perfection to shoot for, then one needs to look at health from a pespective of continuous change. This means that the concept of healthful balance changes. What worked beautifully yesterday may do strange things to our balance today. The concept of health becomes a dynamic motion of input and outflow. If we are to be in constant motion, we can't strive for one balance of health and then nail it down and expect it to be our balance forever.

Flower essences provide a simple and positive framework for identifying periods of change and further identifying changes in our overall balance in light of the new steps forward. Let me give you an example: You are a computer programmer—a very good, highly inventive one who loves your job. For three years your life has felt exciting, comfortable, and pleasing. You have incorporated flower essences into your life and the regular testing verifies your good feelings. You have hardly needed a flower essence during this period. About a month ago, you began to feel fatigued in the evenings. This had never happened before. You test the essences and discover you need Nasturtium Essence. (Restores vital physical life energy during times of intense mental-level focus.) You need to take it for two weeks, two times a day. The definition is saying to you that something in your life has changed that is requiring you to put out more effort on the mental level than your overall balance can maintain. In scanning over your life to find out what is new or where the change has occurred, you remember that about six weeks ago you began work on a project that has required extra focus in order to bring the project to completion. Although the normal pattern of your work has always had its share of high-tension mental activity, something in this particular job has been different and has demanded that you put out just enough to throw off a balance that, up to this point, has worked well for you. Hence the need for Nasturtium Essence.

To continue on the subject of change—that is, anything that requires a shift from the old and familiar to something new, something different. What helps us feel so good and comfortable about the old is that everything in our life, including ourselves, has adjusted to accommodate the old pattern. The more we adjust, the more comfortable we feel. Change includes chaos, or a feeling of chaos. It goes along with the territory. Change requires thinking, adjusting, rearranging, reordering. If a family moves, just the simple chore of finding a grocery store can require a whole lot of thought and effort — certainly more thought and effort than it took to hop in the car and drive the familiar route to the same grocery store for the previous ten years. For kids, changing schools or just starting a new year can add terrific pressures. Or, for adults, a change in work shift, even though the actual job hasn't changed, requires reordering the usual daily schedule. And when one person in a family experiences change, the impact of that change on the others in the family also has to be considered.

As you have probably figured out, I'm not talking about difficult, painful changes in life — although those changes would certainly suggest a need for testing for flower essences too. I'm talking about the normal, good changes, even those changes that are the best thing that ever happened to us. The best change in the world still requires adjustment and reordering on every level of our being. Something as simple as moving from one side of town to another side may mean a change in the drinking water. The body has to get used to this. Or a change in schedule — the body has to get used to this also.

The period of adjustment that accompanies change is unavoidable and can make us vulnerable, sometimes extremely vulnerable. That's when testing for flower essences would be beneficial. The essences won't take away the need for adjustments, but they will stabilize you and allow you to function on all cylinders while you deal with the adjustments. Just being strong, electrically stabilized, and fully present to yourself can do wonders for getting a new life into a new and comfortable order.

I know we can get through these periods of adjustment of which I am speaking without the aid of flower essences. After all, most of us have been doing this quite well for most of our lives. I'm not suggesting that we suddenly create problems where there aren't any and a crutch for that nonexistent problem when no crutch is needed. What I am suggesting falls more into the area of fine-tuning our lives. When the flower essences are tested using kinesiology during different times in our lives, we find out very quickly if essences are needed or not—in other words, if we are holding our balance or not. If the essences aren't needed, all is fine and we are at least assured that we are dealing with this situation with our faculties fully functioning. If our balance has been thrown off and we have flower essences available to us, why in the world would we want to address a situation from an off-balance position? We may be able to slog on through it, and we've all slogged through many times, but why deliberately choose this when we have a chance to do it better? We might surprise ourselves and find out we can handle things a lot better than we thought or previously experienced, if only we gave ourself a break and kept ourselves electrically in balance.

Up to this point, I've really only been addressing the issue of dealing with life more smoothly. I haven't reminded you of the fact that if you allow yourself to remain in a state of imbalance, if you allow the electrical circuitry to remain overloaded or short-circuited, the result will most likely be illness. It's the potential cost of ignoring the times when we overload or short-circuit. Like the cold some people always seem to get at such times. The migrane headache or the shoulder tension or back ache. The touch of depression or constant feeling of low-level fatigue. All those little under-the-weather reactions we tend to accept without question because we've grown accustomed to their being a part of the process. If we are vigilant during times of stress, we can use the flower essences to maintain electrical balance and break the cycle that eventually leads to those adverse physical reactions.

Another time to watch is when we require medical treatments that bring up strong emotional reactions — emotional reactions that we may or may not be expressing outwardly. We're very good at being stoic during these times. I'm referring to things like getting a needle, blood tests, gynecological exams, a visit to your not-so-friendly dentist . . . Recent studies have shown that doctors can't get an accurate blood pressure reading on a lot of their patients because just the fact of being in the doctor's office and being examined is a blood-pressure-raising experience. Also, there's the wait for test results that may confirm our worst fears. Or those hospital stays when we have, as a matter of routine, four injections throughout the day and a battery of tests being done. The more stoic ones tend to translate these times as "being poked and prodded." I recommend that essences be tested before and after an office visit, daily during a waiting period and right after receiving the results, and two or three times a day throughout a hospital stay. Again, it's not a time one should choose to experience from a less than strong position.

Thinking about testing for flower essences during times of trauma is pretty easy, but thinking about them during the times in which we've trained ourselves to ignore the stress and keep plowing through is much more difficult to grasp. Yet it is these times that are more prevalent, and they are the times that tend to lead to the constant pattern of annoying physical reaction. Getting over the resistance to even consider these times as important enough to test for essences is the first hurdle. We really have deeply ingrained resistance about this. It's a part of our good work ethic and our nothing-rattles-me attitude. And to consider, for example, that a change in jobs brought on by a long-awaited promotion could be throwing us off balance to the point where we may develop a cold is obviously a sign of silly self-pampering.

One of my personal challenges while I was learning this was to recognize that when I felt fatigued in any way, it was a sign to sit down right away and test the flower essences. Part of my personal work ethic is to ignore and push on through times of fatigue. I'll rest later. I think a lot of people have similar feelings and reactions. When I tested for essences, I soon found that I always needed something during these times. The fatigue was telling me I had unbalanced. And when I took the essence, I also found that within a few minutes, ten minutes at the most, the feelings of fatigue had totally lifted and I was back to feeling on top of things again. At first, I resisted taking a break from what I was doing. It seemed such a bother and a waste of time. I would argue with myself that I just didn't have time to sit down and test the essences right now. But when I felt the results, it didn't take me long to realize that, by far, the most efficient, time-saving thing to do when I felt a little tired was to stop, test, and take the essence I needed.

What I'm describing to you is a little thing, but it illustrates the change in approach and thinking I'm trying to get across. And it also illustrates how much we can resist even a little change. We can use flower essences during times of illness and trauma, and the essences will serve us well. But to make that shift of awareness, to change how we perceive our balance in relation to the life around us, and to integrate the essences into that change in perception is using flower essences to their fuller potential.

One other thing. When we use the essences to identify moments of imbalance as we move through life, we also identify patterns that could be addressed and changed. Some folks (not many!) can be absolutely fine while going through a dental appointment yet blow about four circuits when faced with seeing a lawyer. The someone who consistently needs an essence whenever they see a lawyer can take that information, look at what it's saying to them, think about their true feelings about seeing a lawyer, and perhaps resolve them, thus breaking this particular pattern. Or they can just identify personal patterns and know that when these arise, they will need the assistance of flower essences.

For example, I met a woman who had been happily married over twenty-five years to a man whose job required that he make two-week trips about four times a year. Every time he took a trip, she got a little cold—nothing big, just a small head cold. By testing her for essences, we found out that her husband's leaving affected her emotionally. She hated to see him leave. Now, that's a fair reaction for someone in love, and she passed the sad feelings off as being silly and never bothered to say anything. But for her, for her sense of balance, these feelings were breaking her electrical circuitry. Through testing, we found out what essences "held" her when she was faced with another trip and separation. We also found out that she needed the essences a full three days prior to her husband's leaving. By clearly identifying the pattern and using the essences accordingly, she was able to maintain balance and stop the pattern of getting head colds. She may or may not be able to address her feelings around these times of separation to the point where she won't need essences at all. But at least she knows what is happening to her, when and how to help herself stay healthy during these times, and what she needs to address if she chooses to alter the pattern.

So, what are my recommendations on how to approach this testing business? I suggest the following guidelines.

1. Definitely test when you are not feeling well. This can mean anything from a slight change in your energy level, to feeling something is coming on, to after you are just plain sick. Concentrate on feeling the subtle warning signs that your body gives as an indication that the balance is now off and your electrical circuitry has shorted. Also anytime when you catch yourself feeling emotionally or mentally low. For example, you realize you are staring at the TV for four hours every night and not caring what you watch or even seeing what you're watching. Or you have no interest in anything going on around you. You can't hold your attention on anything. You just don't give a damn.

2. Test when you are injured or hurt. Test as soon after an accident as possible. I can't tell you the countless burns I've stopped from blistering, the sprains I've stopped from swelling, and the sting reactions I've reversed. An injury is a rapid assault on every level of our being and, most often, our immediate reaction is to either overload or short-circuit. If you want to see vivid evidence of the difference it makes when you use flower essences, treat yourself with essences right after you've been hurt and watch the difference in the healing process. It is amazing to see what we do not need to go through and how fast-paced the recovery and recuperation process can be when the body's electrical circuitry is strong.

3. Test when you are going through obvious change, be it positive or difficult. And maintain the testing throughout the entire period of change and adjustment. Check the kids at the beginning of the school year. Check when there has been a job change or a move to a new home. Check if the family finances suddenly take a nose dive. Or check if the finances have suddenly turned rosy. Some people don't know how to handle success. Test during physical changes such as menopause. And test when there has been a change in relationship: separation, divorce, a child "leaving the nest," the last child *finally* leaving the nest, a friend moving away, the death of someone close, marriage to the person you've been waiting for all of your life, or the birth of a baby.

4. Test when you are going through a therapeutic situation. By this I mean physical, emotional, mental, or spiritual — any situation where you are working with another person for the purpose of making a change, gaining understanding, or improving on something. These frameworks are designed to stir up a great deal. Something as simple as massage, if done correctly, can bring issues to the surface that can suddenly throw us. Flower essences support us as we move through and integrate the process. While in a therapeutic situation, I would suggest testing just prior to each session and right after the session.

5. Check for essences when you are faced with challenge — positive or difficult. A big exam. A major presentation. A speech. An important meeting. A contest. A trial. Any situation where the adrenalin is pumping like crazy. Why not check just prior to see if you are about to enter the challenge on all cylinders?

6. And finally, consider testing yourself daily during the first year of using flower essences. I know this sounds like a major pain in the butt, but once you learn kinesiology it only takes ten seconds to concentrate on the flower essences and test if you need any by asking one question: "Do I need any flower essences?" I suggest this because it is how we uncover those patterns we have so cleverly hidden but that tend to get in our way. It also identifies which situations throw us off balance and which don't. In short, this approach to testing gives us a terrific amount of information about ourselves and how we operate on a day-to-day basis. It teaches us to be more sensitive to ourselves and brings to the surface our individual patterns. After about a year of this kind of fact-finding mission, you probably won't want to stop because you'll see that it really takes no time at all to test daily, and it really keeps you on top of things. But if you should decide to stop the daily testing, by a year's time you should have enough information logged about yourself to enable you to intuitively stay on top of this balance issue.

6

The Basic
Flower Essence Test

Finally comes the moment when you look at all those little bottles and are faced with figuring out which ones you need. As I stated earlier, perhaps the easiest way to choose the flower essences is to look at each bottle and select the one(s) that intuitively attracts your attention. Or you can read down the list of definitions and select the one(s) that jumps out at you. And you can rely on your awareness of your own inner state and choose among the flower essences based on this awareness. These are valid approaches and have been used for years. I know of many practitioners who use one or a combination of the above for discerning which essences their clients need. But the problem I see in this is that the intuitive methods hinge on how clearly and accurately a person's intuition has been developed, and intellectually discerning one's own inner state hinges on the quality and depth with which one is truly able to discern such things at all times.

Another approach that can be quite successful for those who are especially sensitive in the fingertips is to slowly move one or two fingers one-quarter inch above the line of bottles, paying attention to the sensation you feel. Any change in sensation indicates that you need that particular essence. Also, although you are slowly moving the fingers just above the essences, the sensation may be felt elsewhere, like the back of the neck. A person will feel a tingling, or the hair on the back of the neck will "stand up on end." So if this approach appeals to you and you wish to develop it, pay attention to sensation registering anywhere on the body. Refining this takes practice to get it to a point where you can feel confident about using it as a tool.

The best way to discover if you can feel in this manner is to try it — and try it a number of times. It requires that you be very quiet and completely attentive to the process. If you feel any tingling or other sensation, then you can decide if this is what you wish to develop in order to discern the essences. The proof of your accuracy will be the results of your testing plus how you feel after taking those essences. There are many men and women who can feel such things and don't realize it. Again, it's not some psychic trick or magic. It falls into the same domain as some people feeling hot things hotter and cold things colder than others feeling the very same things.

Of course, if you use a pendulum to discern yes/no or positive/negative, you can also use it for the flower essences. Simply move the pendulum over the bottles, and if you are implying the question, "Which ones do I need?" whatever bottles get the positive response are the ones you need.

As you might have guessed already, my personal preference is kinesiology. I like it because it relies on a physical reaction you can feel — your circuit fingers either remain strong or they weaken — and it bypasses the intellect. The intellect is a highly developed and organized framework of knowledge and logic that comes in real handy while one is marching through life. But when dealing with the unknown, the intellect can, and often does, respond as a block. Flower essences often address what we don't consciously know about ourselves, and we can't depend on the intellect to get at the real heart of the issue, only to what we *think* is the heart of the issue. Kinesiology bypasses this. Because it relies on physical reaction, the test tells us emphatically that we either need a specific essence or we don't — no matter what we think. The result is that the input from the flower essences changes our concept of knowledge and logic, and our intellect about such matters becomes more sophisticated.

BASIC TESTING PROCESS

Whatever method you choose for finding out what essences you need, you must approach the testing with clarity and precision. I have set up the following process for kinesiology, but I recommend it for any method.

Prepare for the testing as you would for any kinesiology testing. Choose a quiet room and spend a moment bringing your attention to what you are doing.

1. Place the flower essence bottles in your lap. If they are in a box, you may leave the bottles in the box and place the whole set in your lap. This introduces the essences into your environment.

2. Ask:
Do I need any flower essences? (Test)

If you get a negative result, you're fine. Even though you may be experiencing a situation that sounds like one of the flower essence definitions, your balance is holding and you need no additional assistance. Check again another day to make sure you are still in balance.

3. If the result was positive, you need one or more flower essences. The easiest way to find out which ones is to place the bottles one by one in your lap and ask each time:

Do I need _____ essence? (Test)

The flower essences that test positive are the ones you need. Stand them up in the box or place them to one side to show they tested positive.

4. Check your results by placing in your lap just the bottles that tested positive. Ask:

Are these the only essences I need? (Test)

If the response is positive and you need only one bottle, go on to Step 5.

If you got a negative, retest the other essences. A negative means you missed an essence and need to find what was missed. After retesting, ask the question once more.

Are these the only essences I need? (Test)

If still negative, keep testing the essences until you get a positive response to the question. This will verify to you that you have all the essences you need.

If you have more than one essence, you'll need to check them as a *combination* by placing all of them in your lap and asking:

Is this the combination I need? (Test)

If you get a negative result even though the flower essences tested positive when tested individually, you may need to adjust the combination. This means that when the individual essences that tested positive were put together, a combination was created that made one or more of those essences unnecessary. The whole was stronger and more effective than the sum of its parts. Just test each of the combination bottles separately by asking:

Do I remove this bottle from the combination? (Test)

Whatever tests positive gets removed. Then put the remaining combination bottles in your lap and ask:

Is this combination now correct? (Test)

You should get a positive. If you don't, test the original combination again to find the correct bottle to be removed, and keep working at it until they test positive as a unit.

5. Take the flower essences that you need and read their definitions. The easiest way to take the essences is to put one drop of each essence concentrate on your tongue, being careful not to touch your mouth with the dropper. If you do, wash the dropper well before placing it back in the bottle.

Then ask:

Am I now clear? (Test)

You should test positive at this point, and ninety-eight times out of a hundred, you will. If you test negative, don't panic. You've already double-checked your results, so this test stands as is. A negative result means that you are in need of an additional process. Refer to Chapter 8 under the heading *Peeling* for what to do next.

If you have tested positive for a bunch of essences, let's say ten or more, and after all the double-checking you still test positive for them, take them. I know some folks feel it's not good to take more than three or four at a time, but when using kinesiology you find out precisely what essences make you strong again, reconnect or balance that circuitry, and my feeling is to take what tests positive. I let my body tell me what it needs. If from time to time I break a few established rules about the flower essences, I'll do just that as long as this is what is testing positive for me. This is how I learn both about me and about the flower essences.

However, if you do test positive for a bunch of essences, I will give you one thing to consider. More often than not, I have found that this means a person is structurally out of alignment and needs to see a chiropractor. The essences are temporarily stabilizing the electrical system until the structural alignment is regained. You can easily check this out by asking:

Do I need to see a chiropractor? (Test)

Many chiropractors have incorporated flower essence testing in their practice, and after realigning you, they will test for whatever new essences are needed. If your chiropractor does not use flower essences, be sure to check yourself right after the appointment. (Actually, it would be a good idea to test yourself after any appointment with the chiropractor or any physician.)

Which brings me to another point: using flower essences with medicine. Flower essences do not interfere with medicine and vice versa. If a physician has prescribed medication, continue to take that medication along with the essences. Flower essences are very helpful in the healing process and work well in tandem with needed medication. Remember that by the time you are taking prescribed medication, you are full-fledged into an illness and in need of that support. You are also in need of electrical support and that's where the essences come in. So while you are physically healing with the assistance of medication, you are stabilizing yourself electrically.

One thing to be careful about is testing while you are on medication that makes you drowsy. This will interfere with your ability to hold a focus and even make the testing itself fuzzy. So choose a time when you are your most alert to do the testing. One could say that if the medication makes you drowsy, don't operate heavy machinery or do flower essence testing.

About those medicines we prescribe for ourselves — cold remedies, cough syrup, aspirin, antacids . . . This is the area of medication in which you might consider completely changing over to flower essences. For example, instead of treating a cold with a capsule, treat it with flower essences.

This is where I need to be completely honest with you about myself. Since I began using flower essences — it's been ten years now — I have dealt with all those common household-variety burns, stings, scrapes, sprains, aches, and illnesses using flower essences only. Also, by incorporating essences into my life, I have eliminated the cyclical illnesses we all tend to assume in our lives. In these ten years, I believe I've had a cold two times (I can't think of a third time but I'm not willing to rule out the possibility), and I know I've had the flu only once. In each case, I moved the illness through its cycle very quickly. I had the colds for no more than two days, and the flu that was hitting everyone in our area with a vicious two-week cycle, I got rid of in about eighteen hours. I'm clear on my memory about that because it was New Year's Eve (1983), and Clarence and I had reservations with friends at a fancy restaurant. I woke up that morning with a full-fledged case of the flu, tested for essences every two hours throughout the day, and felt fine, though a little quiet and very much at peace, for the dinner that night. I ate the full meal — all nine courses — and continued to feel fine. Now in the spirit of truth in packaging, I will tell you that I do take two aspirins, two times, on the first day of my menstrual cycle. I do this for two reasons: It's a long-established little habit that I am too lazy to change, and I've heard doctors say that a couple of aspirin periodically help the blood thin and that's supposed to be good. I think it's fair to say that I use the latter as an excuse for the former.

The upshot of what I am trying to say is that if I get sick, I don't reach for any of the stuff they sell in the local drug store; I reach for the flower essences.

I will add one more thing. I try not to be unnecessarily stoic. If I were sick, let's say with a bad cold that I couldn't pull out of, and taking a cold remedy for even a day would give me needed rest, I'd do it. I'd still take the essences, but I'd give myself the break as well. Then I'd back off from the cold remedy as soon as possible and continue on with the essences. I personally have not gotten into that situation yet, but this would be a course of action I'd consider and something I wouldn't hesitate suggesting to someone else.

Also, I do not suggest that flower essences replace physicians — not completely. As you have seen from my own medical history these past ten years, physicians and across-the-counter drug manufacturers do not get rich from me. I urge common sense around this issue of physician vs. flower essences. There are times when our condition warrants a strong, multidirectional approach, and this is where the physician comes in. I'm well aware that this is an emotional issue with some people. I can't resolve this issue for you since it's a matter of personal choice. All I can say is that for those of you who don't wish to use mainstream medical help, you're going to love what the essences can do for you. For those of you who do see physicians, you're going to love the drastically reduced number of office visits and fewer medical expenses.

Back to the testing: The steps I gave for testing are very deliberate and precise, and are designed to verify your test results and catch errors all along the way. In the beginning, while getting used to it, I recommend you stick to this approach. When you feel confident about your testing and your ability to focus well, you'll see ways to move more quickly through the process without losing "quality control." For example, you can keep the whole set in your lap, touch each bottle with a free finger, and test down the line, one bottle at a time. Or you can keep the box in your lap and simply read the name of each essence, keeping your attention on that specific bottle, and test down the line, one bottle at a time. One warning about reading the names this way: It is inevitable that as we grow accustomed to testing, we begin to get a little sloppy. One of the first things to watch out for is the practice we have of saying to ourselves one word, the word we've just read, while at the same time focusing our attention on the next word we want to read. For example, you are asking if you need Gruss an Aachen while, at the same time, you are looking at the label on the next bottle, Peace. You've just divided your focus, and in reality, your electrical system doesn't really know if you are asking about Gruss an Aachen or Peace, and you'll get a weak, weird-feeling test result.

For both kinesiology and the flower essences to function at their highest, it is vital that you keep your focus on precisely what you are asking and testing. The act, although cumbersome and time-consuming, of placing one bottle at a time in your lap eliminates a lot of the potential areas for split focus. That's why I recommend it until you feel comfortable about testing—which includes feeling comfortable about your ability to maintain focus.

To give you an idea of the time involved in testing, I'd say that in the very beginning you'll be spending about 20 to 30 minutes testing a set of eighteen flower essences like the Perelandra Garden Essences. This includes going through all the steps slowly and cranking your fingers equally as slowly—as it should be in the beginning. Very quickly, after you begin testing and get the hang of what it all feels like, it will take you about 10 to 15 minutes to test eighteen essences. Now, I don't mean to sound like I'm boasting (after all, you must remember I've been doing essence testing a lot over the past ten years), but to give you an idea of how quickly all those steps I've given you can be done, it takes me no more than two minutes to do an entire test readout on myself. So if everything feels cumbersome and too damned time-consuming in the beginning, just have a little patience. It'll smooth out with practice.

TESTING FOR DOSAGE

This is to find out how many days or weeks you are to take the essences you just tested for.

1. Hold all the bottles you need in your lap.

2. Ask if you need to take the flower essence(s) more than one time. If negative, that means, "No, you don't need to take them more than one time," and you have already completed the essence test by putting one drop from each bottle on your tongue.

(Again, be careful not to touch your mouth with the dropper. If you touch the dropper, wash it well before putting it back into the bottle so that the flower essence won't be contaminated. Children are especially talented at getting that dropper!)

3. If positive, you will need to find out how many days you should have the flower essences and how many times per day. This is easy. Use kinesiology again. With the needed flower essence(s) in your lap, ask yourself:

Do I need these 1 day? (Test)

2 days? (Test)

3 days? (Test)

Do a sequential count until you get a negative response. If you need the flower essences for 3 days, you will test positive when you ask, "1 day?", "2 days?", "3 days?" When you ask, "4 days?" you will test negative. That will tell you that your system is assisted and strengthened by the flower essences for 3 days, not 4 days.

HINT: If you are testing sequentially and you get positive responses up to 14 days, switch your approach and test sequentially in weeks rather than days. This little trick will save wear and tear on the testing fingers. Just ask:

Do I need them for 2 weeks? (Test)

3 weeks? (Test)

4 weeks? (Test)

And so on until you get a negative. Let's say you get a negative on 5 weeks. That means you need them for 4 weeks. Now ask:

Do I need them for more than 4 weeks? (Yes)

4 weeks plus 1 day? (Yes)

4 weeks plus 2 days? (Yes)

4 weeks plus 3 days? (No)

You need to take these essences for a total of 4 weeks plus 2 days.

DAILY DOSAGE

Let's say you test that you need to take the flower essences for 3 days. Now using the same format, ask if you should take the essences:

    1 time daily? (Test)

    2 times daily? (Test)

And so on, until you get a negative. Most people need to take them either 1 or 2, sometimes 3, times a day. Test until you get a negative response. Your last positive will tell you how many times per day you need to take them.

Generally, flower essences are to be taken first thing in the morning and/or last thing in the evening and/or in the mid-afternoon. If you wish to be more precise with this essence business, test to see if it is best to take them in the morning, afternoon, or evening, or any combination of the three. For example, if I am testing someone who tests for a dosage of one time a day, I always check to see if it should be in the morning, afternoon, or evening. It is usually in the morning, but I've discovered enough exceptions to that rule to test every time.

For dosages of a number of essences taken several times throughout the day over a period of days, it may be more convenient to add 9 drops of each needed essence to 4 ounces of water (spring water or distilled water is preferred). Take one sip from this mixed solution each time you are to take the flower essences. (It is more effective if you hold the sip of solution in your mouth for a few seconds prior to swallowing.) You can store the mixture in the refrigerator, or preserve it by adding 3 teaspoons of brandy or distilled white vinegar. If the glass is emptied before you are scheduled to finish taking the essences, just make the same preparation again.

HINT: You can test for the precise number of drops of each essence to go into the 4 ounces of water if you like. Just use the same sequential setup as was used to discover the dosage. For each essence, ask:

Do I need 1 drop per 4 ounces of water? (Test)

2 drops? (Test)

3 drops? (Test)

And so on until you get a negative. This testing economizes to the utmost on the use of your concentrates. I've suggested you use 9 drops per 4 ounces of water because in my experience, I've never tested anyone for over 9 drops (most people test an average of 3 drops), and I figure right about now you'd appreciate a break in this testing routine.

DOSAGE BOTTLES

You need several essences several times a day, you work away from the home all day, and it's real cumbersome to transport a glass of water everywhere. No problem. Your local pharmacy sells one-ounce or one-half-ounce dropper bottles. Buy a couple to keep on hand. Make the solution as needed right in the bottle, adding 5 drops of each essence to a one-half-ounce bottle and filling the rest of the bottle with water. If you are planning to use this bottle for more than a couple of days, add one teaspoon of brandy as a preservative (use more if the essences are to be taken for longer than two weeks or are exposed to high temperatures) before filling with water. Shake the dosage bottle lightly.

Several flower essences may be combined in one bottle. In fact, however many flower essences test positive for each solution may be combined in one bottle. One dropper full, about 10 to 12 drops, from the dosage bottle can be put directly into the mouth. (Again, be careful not to touch the mouth with the dropper.)

A note on the water to be used in these solutions: Spring or untreated water is best. But if this is unavailable, tap water will suffice. You can also refrigerate the solution.

One last thing: There is a question of whether flower essences from one set should be mixed with flower essences from another set. I let kinesiology answer that for me. If I test for three essences, two from the Perelandra sets and one from another, I simply test whether it is alright to combine them into one solution. If I get a positive result, I mix them. And I tell others that if the Perelandra flower essences test to be mixed with other essences, by all means do it.

A reminder: If you are sensitive to brandy, you may use *distilled white vinegar* as a brandy substitute for preserving your solution. Use the same amount of vinegar as you would brandy for proper preservation. Also, you can dilute the concentrates, nine drops in four ounces of water, and the brandy will be tasteless.

FOLLOW-UP TESTING

Often the completion of a situation or process we might be involved in will require a series of flower essences. For example, after doing the basic test, you found that you needed two essences for three days, two times a day. On the day following the completion of this dosage, retest for essences to find out if a new dosage is needed. You may discover that you now need one essence for two days, one time a day. Once this is completed, test again. Keep doing this testing each time you have completed a dosage cycle until you test that no other essences are needed. This means that you are clear, and that either the process or situation has now completed or your balance is holding well as you move through the remainder of the cycle.

The issue of follow-up testing is vital to the successful use of flower essences. Frequently I find that people are willing to do the first test, especially when they are not feeling well. They take the needed essences as prescribed and rave about how much better they feel. Then they don't do the follow-up testing, and often the result is that they slip right back into feeling lousy. Just as there are stages in the recuperation period, there are corresponding stages in the flower essences needed. And sometimes the lousy feelings may be completely gone and we think we have come to the end, but we still test the need for essences. This just means we're still in the recuperation period and, despite all evidence to the contrary, it hasn't ended yet. In short, it's important to follow through with the essence testing all the way to the end.

One other thing to caution you about: Let's say you just got rid of a bad cold. You did all the follow-up testing and you finally tested clear—no other essences needed. Everything is going well for about five days and then you start to feel the cold coming back. As soon as you get those first signs, go right back to testing the essences. This does not mean you made an error in the previous series of tests. Most likely it means that something unexpected has happened in your life and, while in that vulnerable period right after being sick, it just broadsided you, breaking or overloading your electrical circuitry again. If you move quickly with the essences, you'll reestablish the balance and prevent getting sick again. However, if you do get sick again, keep testing the essences as you move through it until you test clear.

KEEPING RECORDS

This is for the people who want to find out more about themselves. Keep a record of the date, the illness or situation, the symptoms you feel, and the essences needed plus dosage. This is especially helpful during that first year or so of using the essences. Eventually you'll be able to look over the record and see what reactions and types of situations result in what symptoms — what situation tends to be the underlying cause of our headaches, or our lower backache, or the sinus trouble. It's another way of discovering personal patterns. If we know that whenever we got a sinus headache we tended to need Zinnia Essence (Reconnects one to the child within. Restores playfulness, laughter, joy, and a sense of healthy priorities.), we can reexamine our life in light of the priorities we choose and our somber attitude, and make some changes that would strike a better balance for us. This would then break the personal patterning that results in sinus headaches. So besides using flower essences to pull us out of each sinus headache, we can use them to begin eliminating the sinus headache cycle altogether.

The following are the basic testing steps in a condensed form for easy reference while you are doing the testing.

BASIC TESTING STEPS

1. Prepare to test and place the flower essences in your lap.

2. Ask:
   Do I need any flower essences? (Test)

3. If positive, test each bottle separately. Stand the bottles up in the box or set aside the ones that test positive.

4. Place in your lap the bottles that test positive and ask,
   Are these the only essences I need? (Test)

If the response is positive and you need only one bottle, go on to Step 5.

If negative, you've missed one/some and need to retest the other essences. Place the new ones in your lap along with the ones that already tested positive and ask again,
   Are these the only essences I need? (Test)

If the response is negative, you're still missing an essence. Keep retesting the other essences until you get a positive response to the question. (If you're getting all kinds of crazy responses with bottles sometimes testing positive, sometimes negative, you're nervous. Put all the bottles back in the box, walk around the room or take a short break, then come back to the essences and start from the beginning. Concentrate on the testing and not on the doubts you might have from the previous testing experience.)

Once you test positive to the question and you need more than one bottle, you have a combination. Place the bottles in your lap and ask:
   Is this the combination I need? (Test)

If negative, adjust the combination by removing unnecessary essences. That is, test each bottle separately by asking,

Is this bottle needed in the combination? (Test)

Remove the bottles that test negative and check the new combination by asking:

Is this combination now correct? (Test)

Continue working with the combination until it tests positive.

5. Test for dosage: Do the sequential testing to discover the number of days needed, number of times per day, and time(s) of day to be taken. Test for the number of drops needed for the solution, or use 5 drops of each essence per one-half-ounce dropper bottle, or 9 drops of each per 4 ounces of water.

6. Take the flower essences you tested for and *read their definitions*. Then ask:

Am I now clear? (Test)

If negative, refer to Chapter 8, *Peeling* section.

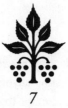

7

Surrogate Testing

IT'S REALLY HELPFUL FOR THOSE who are interested in incorporating flower essences in their life to learn to use them for themselves. So much information is available through essence use, and using essences well is quite a simple matter. But there are situations and times when it is appropriate for us to do the testing for another who, for whatever reason, is unable to test for himself. This is especially true with children, someone who is ill, a troubled friend, or just someone who needs essences from time to time and doesn't want to learn to test for themselves.

You can help in these situations by testing that person in the same manner you have learned to test for yourself by using a kinesiology surrogate technique. If you are developing a flower essence testing technique other than kinesiology, I suggest you still set up your session with the person in much the same manner as I describe in order to maintain the precision and clarity required for accurate testing.

1. *Test yourself first.* Take any needed flower essences to make sure you are clear before testing anyone else.

This step is vital. If you attempt to test someone while you are in need of essences yourself, what *you* need will test as an essence the other person needs. Rather than you reading him, he is picking up on you. This often is graphically demonstrated in workshops I have given where I have a number of people verifying the testing of another person who is testing himself. As this person tests each essence, the five or six others will be surrogate testing him as a verification. Invariably, one of the surrogate testers will forget to clear himself, and for one essence, everyone but this individual (surrogate tester #3) will test that it is not needed for the person doing the primary testing. Surrogate tester #3 keeps testing positive, it's needed. Then I'll suggest that #3 test himself, and always the essence in question is the one he needs. He'll take it, resume his role as surrogate tester, retest the essence in question, and now everyone gets a negative.

Surrogate testing by definition requires the interaction of two people. Ideally the tester is open to and reading the electrical strengths and weaknesses of the person being tested. If the tester himself is not clear, as far as the essences are concerned, and focused on the testing, he will either not be connected properly to the other person and simply be reading a test from himself, or the roles will reverse and the tester's needs will blend into the system of the other person and those needs, in turn, will be registering as the weaknesses of the one being tested. This phenomenon doesn't just occur with flower essences testing. Physicians using kinesiology to discern which vitamins a patient needs will run into the same situation. If the physician's system needs vitamin B_6, the person he is testing will also show a need for vitamin B_6. The only way to insure that the test results you are getting in surrogate testing are from the person you are testing is to make sure you are clear, that is, not in need of the thing you are testing for—in this case, flower essences.

2. Physically make contact with the person you are going to test. For example, have them place a hand on your knee or touch your foot with their foot. Let the person know that they must keep their mind on the testing and not let their mind idly wander from thought to thought, or to last night's hockey score. This will cause fuzzy or inaccurate testing results. To help them stay focused, tell them to watch what you are doing. Also, it may help to give them something to listen to, so talk to them about the process as you move through it. If you are testing a small child, you can usually keep them focused on the testing by moving the boxes and bottles around a lot and engaging them in a little conversation about what's going on. If it's impossible for them to focus, plan to test them while they're asleep. However, for infants, I find that I have no problems testing them whether they are asleep, awake, crying or not. As long as I can maintain my concentration, the testing moves smoothly.

Concentrate your focus on the person for a few seconds. The physical touching and focus connects their electrical system to yours. Test your connection using the kinesiology technique, asking (aloud or to yourself):

Am I fully connected to this person's electrical system?
(Test)

If negative, spend a few more seconds focusing on the individual. If either of you is being distracted, move to a quieter room or quiet the environment you are in. Encourage the other person to keep their mind on the test.

If you have a parent with a child and you are trying to test the parent, the child must be on its own elsewhere in the room and occupied in order for the parent to have full attention on the testing. The child cannot be sitting on the parent's lap. Also the child cannot be sitting on the parent's lap if you are testing the child. You'll need to take care that the physical systems of parent and child, or child and sibling, are independent from one another. This situation usually occurs when working with parent and child, but it is a good practice to always make sure the person you are testing is physically detached from everyone else in the vicinity, like well-meaning spouses or friends who want to give support by holding the person's hand.

3. If the test for your connection to the other person was positive, you are ready to test for the flower essences. Place the bottles (or box of bottles) *in your lap* and ask:

Does he/she need any of these flower essences? (Test)

If the result is negative, nothing in their electrical circuitry is broken and they are fine. You can double-check your result by asking the question over and retesting. If it is still negative, the testing is over.

If positive, place each bottle, one at a time, *in your lap* and ask:

Is _____ flower essence needed? (Test)

You don't have to say these things out loud, and for each bottle you can shorten the question to "This one?" A positive test response indicates that this particular flower essence balances the other person's system and makes it strong. They need it.

Double-check your results by placing all the needed bottles in the free hand or lap *of the person* and ask again:

Are these all the flower essences needed? (Test)

If negative, first make sure your connection with this person is still positive. Ask:

Am I fully connected to this person's electrical system? (Test)

If you weren't, go back to the connection process in Step 2 and do the testing over again.

If the connection was fine, retest the other essences to find what was missed. Ask again:

Are these the essences needed? (Test)

If the response is positive and only one bottle is needed, go on to Step 4.

If negative, you're still missing an essence. Keep retesting the other essences until you get a positive response to the question.

For a combination, place the combination bottles *in the person's* free hand or lap and ask:

Is this the combination he/she needs? (Test)

If negative, adjust the combination by removing any unnecessary essences. Test each bottle separately by having the person hold it, and asking:

Is this bottle needed in the combination? (Test)

Whatever tests negative gets removed. Check the new combination by asking:

Is this combination now correct? (Test)

HINT: When testing a baby, the bottles need only be placed on or right next to the child.

I usually find we operate better when we understand why we're doing what we're doing. So I'll explain a little about why I set this step up the way I did. There are a number of ways you can do the actual testing of the flower essences with another person. You can test without the essences themselves being touched by you or the person you are testing. All you have to do is read down the row of labels or a list of the names. Or you can go the other way and have the person you are testing touch each essence as you test your own circuit fingers. As a matter of clarity, I have you as the tester doing the testing and making physical contact with the essences — going that extra step to make sure you have control of the testing.

Hopefully by the time you do surrogate testing you will have developed enough discipline to really focus on what you are doing. You'll have worked with all those pitfalls around kinesiology, or at least know what to watch out for. The more the other person becomes involved in the testing technique itself, the more chance they have of falling into those pitfalls. Usually, I find it is quite enough for them to simply keep their mind from wandering throughout the testing. So I've set all of this up in order to keep as much of the actual testing technique in the control of the surrogate tester as possible.

SOME SITUATIONS TO WATCH OUT FOR DURING THE TESTING:

A. If you are testing a parent whose child is in the room and the child calls out, the parent's mind will immediately shift from the testing to the child. Stop the testing and wait until the parent is ready to refocus. Then continue where you left off.

B. Sometimes the testing is boring to the person because nothing is being felt or said — especially if you are in the learning stages of testing and it's going slowly. If they let their mind wander, you'll begin to feel fuzzy test results. Or you'll start getting what essences they need when they are driving to work, or trying to figure out when to do the grocery shopping, or thinking about their last date. What you want to do is keep their attention on the testing. One easy trick is to say out loud everything you are doing and the names of all the essences you are testing as you go along. That way they don't get lost in the quiet.

C. If anything should happen around you during the testing that pulls the person's attention away—like a phone ringing, a car backfiring, a siren in the distance, the child dropping a book— allow both of you the few seconds needed to focus back on the testing. Don't try to plow through a distraction.

D. Also, if you are having trouble focusing, don't hesitate to stop the testing and rectify the situation. When I'm doing surrogate testing, I am continuously reminded how little people understand what is going on and the operating principles behind kinesiology—even after I've told them what I'm doing and why. More often than not, the responsibility for setting up the environment for the testing is left up to me—and will be left up to you. Flower essence testing will usually be done by you in an informal environment rather than an office environment. Don't be surprised if after telling someone you'll need a little quiet in order to test them for essences, they turn around and scream to the four-teen-year-old to turn down his boom box but say nothing about the TV volume or the teapot that is about to boil over at any minute. Now, silencing the boom box may be just the kind of quiet that person needs in order to focus. Some people, especially parents, numb themselves to racket and chaos as a survival technique. But if you as the tester are not able to maintain focus throughout an entire testing process with this kind of racket, you must take the initiative and suggest a move to another room. On the other hand, if you're doing fine in this situation but you notice the person you are testing is glancing over your shoulder to watch what's happening on TV, you need to eliminate the distraction and corral this person's focus back to the testing.

Usually the situation isn't this obvious. You'll just have to be careful about two things: your own needs for giving a good test and what you need to do to assist the other person's focus. In time, as you get more comfortable with testing for yourself and others, you'll be able to do this kind of thing in the middle of the annual Christmas office party, if necessary.

4. When the needed flower essences have been determined, test for how many days/weeks and how many times a day, using the same sequential testing procedure you use on yourself. It is important that you remain physically connected with the other person throughout the entire testing process.

5. Give the needed essences to the person. This can be either one drop of each essence concentrate or a solution mixed in a glass of water. Once taken, ask:

Is this person now clear? (Test)

You should get a positive, especially after all the double-checking you did throughout. If, on a rare occasion, you should get a negative, the person may need an additional process. Refer to Chapter 8 under the heading *Peeling*.

HINTS: When giving essences to an infant up to three months old, you may place a drop of the essence concentrate directly onto the forehead and, with your finger, lightly rub the essence into the skin. This is one way to bypass giving an infant brandy. For an older child who may protest the taste of brandy or vinegar, make a solution of their essences in a 4-ounce glass of water. This will dilute the concentrate enough to make it tasteless. For a child under 12 years of age, just add one drop of each essence to four ounces of water. The child does not have to drink the entire 4 ounces to receive the proper dosage. In fact, only 3 gulps are needed.

If flower essences are needed for a period of time, mix the drops in a glass of water (9 drops per 4 ounces of water for an adult, or test for number of drops of each essence needed) or fix a dosage bottle. Be sure to add brandy or distilled vinegar if the essences are to be used for more than a couple of days. The dosage can be stored in the refrigerator without adding a preservative. Remind them to wash the dropper before sticking it back into the bottle if they touch it with their tongue.

6. It is important that you explain how, when, and how long to take the essences. It is also important that they know which essences they are taking and what the definitions are. At least let them read the definitions. Better yet, have them copy the short definitions of the essences they need so that they can refer back to them later. Also, schedule for follow-up testing, if needed.

HINT: You may experience a hunger attack after surrogate testing. This usually occurs when you have surrogate tested a number of people in a row and have been required to maintain a sharp focus on the testing over an extended period of time. In order to hold the focus you have used protein – this is normal for maintaining strong focus – and your body's protein level has become spent. So, if you feel hungry after a testing period, immediately eat something high in protein. As you become more used to the focus required for surrogate testing, you'll notice that the post-testing hunger attack will occur less often. If, however, it doesn't lessen for you, plan to eat something high in protein prior to any long testing period. This will stabilize you during the testing and you won't use up your protein reserves.

The most common question that comes up when talking about surrogate testing, and personal testing, for that matter, has to do with the possibility of making a mistake. Luckily, here's where the beauty of the flower essences really shines. You can't overdose the system with the essences. Either your electrical circuitry is connected and balanced or it isn't. The wrong essence doesn't short-circuit or overload a balanced system or short-circuit an already weakened system in new ways. When you take a flower essence that you don't need, the body simply throws off the essence. People who see vibrational color have reported seeing an unneeded essence enter the body's auric field as a color, then become enveloped by another color emanating from the body, and be moved completely out of the auric field. In short, the body rejects an unnecessary flower essence.

Where you could get into trouble is the input of information through the definitions. If you've made a mistake, the information the faulty definition gives may confuse the person or detour their process. But I have found that the person is more likely to intellectually throw off the information in much the same manner as the body throws off the actual essence energy. They simply won't be able to recall the information or they'll be a complete blank about the whole testing experience.

Lastly, the same thing applies around the issue of flower essences and medicine in surrogate testing, as in using the essences for yourself. Flower essences do not supercede medicines and vice versa, nor does either interfere with the other.

THE ETHICAL ISSUE

Each of us has to make up our mind as to how we approach others regarding flower essences. They are gentle, easy, effective — but powerful. Because of their nature, they address the heart or cause of an issue rather than the results. And because of this, I do not test someone unless *they* ask me. I feel they must give me permission to, in effect, enter their privacy. I also feel that they know their own timing, consciously or unconsciously, and I can't know that for them.

If I see someone who I feel would benefit from the flower essences and he doesn't know anything about them, I will tell him what the essences are, what, in my experience, they do, and how they work. Then I will say that if he feels comfortable about this, I will be very happy to test him for flower essences. I urge him to use his intuition or gut feelings as to whether or not he wants the test. If he has any hesitation, I back right off. I do not feel he is saying something negative about me or the flower essences; rather he is indicating to me, as master of his own dance, that it is not appropriate just yet.

If someone is unconscious and therefore unable to make a decision (these people, as will be explained in Chapter 8, can be tested exactly as you would any surrogate testing), I feel that I as the tester must assume a role and responsibility in the decision making. I don't go charging in dispensing essences because I know these things are good and helpful. The fact that they are good and helpful, to me, is beside the point. The issue is whether or not they are to be used for this person at this time. For that decision, I try my best to come up with the best intuitive answer in light of the other person, not based on my emotional desire to help. If I know the person already has used flower essences, that tells me it's a safe bet they'd like the essences used in this instance. If they haven't used them before and you have time (they are in a coma in the hospital), you can talk to them, literally, about the essences, explaining everything exactly as you would if they were conscious. Then connect with them physically, touch their arm or hand, and ask *them* if they wish for you to use the essences. Test using kinesiology, and go with your answer. If there is no time for all this talking and testing, but there's opportunity to use the essences, I'd have to go with my intuition as to what that person wants and accept the responsibility for that decision.

THE SURROGATE TESTING STEPS

1. *Test and clear yourself first.*

2. Physically make contact with the person and make sure their attention is on the testing. And you focus on them for a few seconds. Test your connection:

Am I fully connected to this person's electrical system? (Test)

3. Place the flower essences *in your lap* and ask (aloud or to yourself):

Does he/she need any of these essences? (Test)

If positive, test each bottle. Pull out the bottles that test positive. Double-check by placing the bottles testing positive *into the person's* free hand or lap. Ask:

Are these all the essences needed? (Test)

If negative, double-check your connection with this person:

Am I fully connected to _____'s electrical system? (Test)

If not, go back to Step 2, refocus on the person, and do the testing over again.

If you are connected, retest the other essences to find what was missed. Ask again:

Are these all the essences needed? (Test)

If the response is positive and only one bottle is needed, go on to Step 4.

If negative, you're still missing an essence. Keep retesting the other essences until you get a positive response to the question.

For a combination, place the combination bottles *in the person's* free hand or lap, and ask:

Is this the combination he/she needs? (Test)

If negative, adjust the combination by removing any unnecessary essences. Test each bottle separately by having the person hold it and asking:

Is this bottle needed in the combination? (Test)

Whatever tests negative gets removed. Check the new combination by asking:

Is this combination now correct? (Test)

Continue working with the combination until it tests positive.

4. Remaining physically connected with the person, test for how many days/weeks and how many times per day the essences need to be taken. Use 5 drops of each essence concentrate per one-half-ounce bottle, or 9 drops of each per 4 ounces water.

5. Administer the flower essences needed either directly on the tongue or in a glass of water. Test to make sure the person is now clear. (Refer to Chapter 8, section on *Peeling* if they are not.) For

flower essences to be taken more than one time: Mix the drops in a glass of water or fix a dosage bottle. Add brandy or distilled vinegar as a preservative if the solution is to be kept unrefrigerated.

6. Explain when, how, and how long to take the essences. Explain which flower essences they needed and let them read and/or copy the definitions. Schedule for follow-up testing, if needed.

8

Additional Flower Essence Procedures

THE BASIC FLOWER ESSENCE TESTING PROCESS can be used as a starting point for a number of additional procedures I've developed to address specific issues in a clear and exact manner. If flower essences in general get to the heart of issues, these additional procedures are designed to get to the very center point of that heart. Including them, when needed, allows you to work the essences with the highest of efficiency and precision.

I am presenting these procedures for you to use as an individual testing yourself. They all can be expanded for surrogate testing exactly as the basic testing has been expanded.

Important: Before doing any of these procedures, it is imperative that you do the basic essence test first. They are to be in addition to the basic test, not in place of it. The basic test balances you in an overall, general manner and you must be "cleared" generally in order to use these more precise procedures.

Also, reading about these procedures the first time, you may feel completely overwhelmed. Don't get discouraged. Just put these additional procedures aside and concentrate on developing the basic test first. Then when you feel less overwhelmed, work on incorporating the procedures one at a time as you need them.

PEELING

I call this procedure "peeling" because it reminds me of the many layers of an onion. Essentially what happens here is that you have gone through the basic testing process, selected and taken the correct flower essences, and have asked the question, "Am I clear?" Much to your surprise, you got a negative test result to the question. This indicates that you are in a peeling process. That is, whatever is making you feel unwell or unbalanced is in layers, and when you took the first essences, you peeled away the first layer, allowing the second layer to be exposed or to rise to the surface. (I know I'm mixing my metaphors here, but both concepts accurately describe what this phenomenon feels like.)

Sometimes something hits us that we consciously or unconsciously do not wish to look at or deal with. Usually we are afraid of the issue itself or the possible outcome in which it might result. It doesn't stop us from being hit by the issue. So what we do immediately is hide the issue under a layer formed by a related issue that is less threatening. And being the emotionally and mentally complex individuals that we are, we hide that layer with another less intense but related issue. This process can go on until we have a top layer that on the surface looks to be nothing. Taken on its own, it is nothing. But in this case, the surface layer is serving to shield us from everything layered beneath it. The whole thing, the entire onion, eventually becomes too much for us to handle and we physically begin to feel the pressure. If ignored long enough, we'll feel downright emotionally or physically sick. So we respond by testing the essences, and without our realizing it, the first test gets rid of the top layer. The negative answer to the question, "Am I clear?" just indicated you are not. Something else has been exposed.

At this point, I would suggest you write down the essences you took for the first test and continue recording the essences you need for the rest of the process. This will come in handy later when you want to look at the core issue and how you hid it from yourself.

Do the basic process again. This test addresses the second layer only. Take those essences and ask again if you are clear. If you get another negative, you've uncovered a third layer. Do the basic process again, addressing the third layer. Take those essences, and ask the question. It's important that you keep your focus on the layer you are testing and not try to figure out the previous layer or anticipate the next layer. Continue doing this until you get a positive to the question, "Am I clear?" Each time you get a negative to the question, don't bother doing any dosage tests (number of days, etc.) because all you are doing is addressing layers for the purpose of getting them out of the way in order to uncover the next layer. The essences for each layer are needed one time only during the peeling procedure. When you finally ask if you are clear and get a positive, you have reached the central issue and that's when you need to do a dosage test.

Usually I have found that it takes the removal of about three or four layers before hitting the central issue. However, I have worked with people where I had to deal with fifteen to twenty layers before getting to the real issue at hand. You need to keep going until you test positive on being clear.

Also, I have found that as I'm working with peeling, the results from the test for one layer tend not to have any logical connection with the results for the next layer. But quite often, once we get to the core issue and see those test results, the other essences finally begin to make sense. Even if they don't make complete sense or don't seem logically connected to one another, we can still look at what is being indicated with each layer and learn what precisely we tend to do to create the layers. This is where keeping a record of the essences needed for each layer is helpful. We can identify patterns of behavior or reaction that, when observed down the road, can serve to tip us off that we may be creating an onion, and testing flower essences would stop the process.

You may get all the way to the core issue and still have absolutely no idea what the specific issue is that caused the building of layers in the first place. Don't fret. Just take those final essences for the prescribed amount of time, and I guarantee you that at some point in the near future, while you're riding the A-Train to work, watching a football game, or just basically doing nothing, it'll hit. Don't forget that the reason you created the onion in the first place was because something was very difficult for you to look at and you blew a circuit or two or three. While you are taking the essences, the circuits have been reconnected and balanced, and you are being supported and stabilized, thus making it possible for this issue to come into your awareness. Once you figure out what happened, you will probably see that something has to be faced or dealt with. I suggest you stay close to the flower essences while you go through this process. You already know that in this issue your pattern is to hide the situation as deeply as possible. Frequent testing for the need for essences keeps what is important on the surface, keeps you stabilized and functioning on all cylinders as you deal with the issue, and keeps the onion from forming again.

One other thing—don't underestimate the intensity and impact of the core issue. Sometimes we can get hit with the awareness of what it is and say to ourselves, "You've got to be kidding. Is that all it is?" At this point, we are judging the issue from the standpoint of logic and what we think is acceptable stress. Anything less than acceptable stress is akin to babying and coddling ourself. The peeling procedure tells us that despite what we think and no matter what our value judgment is regarding such matters, this particular issue is so threatening to us that we had to try to cover it with layer upon layer. If you can't believe that such an insignificant issue could cause all of this, yet you are interested in breaking the patterns that cause you to create onions when faced with this or similar issues, you really need to sit down and think about it as honestly and completely as possible in order to understand what's the real problem here.

Steps for the Peeling Process

1. Do this process immediately after it is indicated for in the basic essence test. Just remain focused and move right into the peeling process.

2. Do another basic test. Take those essences. Keep a record of the ones you need.

3. Ask:
   Am I now clear? (Test)

If positive, go on to Step 5.

4. If negative, repeat Steps 2 and 3 until you get a positive response to the question.

5. The essences that test positive in the final test are the ones that are directly related to the core issue. Read their definitions. Test for number of days needed and times per day you are to take them.

6. Do any necessary follow-up testing once the prescribed dosage period ends. This will support you during the period of insight and integration that will follow the peeling process.

TELEGRAPH TESTING

The telegraphing procedure is an important tool to develop and have at hand. It allows you to use flower essences with pinpoint accuracy, and I have found that when dealing with specific symptoms, and by using telegraphing along with the basic testing procedure, you can move through some symptoms with lightning speed — minutes instead of hours or days.

I'll give you an example of how this works and then I'll tell you why it works. Let's say you were working out in the backyard doing some spring cleaning and you got stung on the hand by a wasp. Hurt like hell. Being the wise individual that you are, you immediately stopped what you were doing, pulled the stinger out, came into the house, and tested for flower essences. According to the results of the basic test, you needed Broccoli Essence, Yellow Yarrow and Gruss an Aachen. You put a drop from each of these on your tongue. You felt a change, perhaps even a strengthening right after you took these essences, but you did not feel any discernable difference in the sting symptoms. Now, the basic test addresses your balance within the context of your complete body environment. In other words, it addresses the large picture. Telegraphing addresses one issue — in this case it would address just the wasp sting. So, to continue the scenario, after taking Broccoli, Yellow Yarrow and Gruss an Aachen, you placed your full focus on the sting (due to the pain, this wasn't too hard!) and tested all the essences again while maintaining that focus. In short, you tested the sting itself. This time you found the need for Tomato and Yellow Yarrow. Keeping your focus on the sting, you took both Tomato and Yellow Yarrow. Instantaneously, the pain decreased dramatically and the redness visibly diminished, and within about ten minutes, the swelling began to go down.

Now, let me explain how and why this worked. I call this procedure "telegraphing" because a direct linkup is made to something specific through the use of focus. There are several principles of energy involved here. 1) To move energy from point A to point B, one need only utilize visualization or focus to accomplish that move. 2) To *link* point A to point B, all one needs to do is visualize that link or focus with the intent of creating the link, and the necessary energy will shift in order to accommodate the focus and accomplish the link. 3) Energy can easily be modified through the use of visualization or focus. 4) Energy precedes form. Therefore, to impact one form (form A) with another (form B), one need only introduce into form A the energy of form B, and the physical properties of form B will shift into form A, thus impacting and altering it.

When I use the word "focus," I'm talking about the kind of attention it takes to listen to someone tell you something important at 2:30 in the afternoon on the floor of the New York Stock

Exchange. If you are following every word this person is saying, you are focused on that person and getting the full impact of what is being told to you. If you hear that person but at the same time you are aware of the commotion going on around you, you're not focused. At best, you're half-listening. In telegraphing, the focus on a specific area or symptom is to such a degree that, for the moment, nothing else within your body environment is attracting your attention. When this occurs, an electrical link is created, very similar to the electrical line linking two ends within a telegraph system — only the line in the body is created by the energy and intent of the focus and is not physically discernable.

When telegraph testing, you are not testing that one thing in relationship to the whole. That you did when you did the basic test procedure. Instead, you are testing the one thing on its own in relationship to nothing else. Consequently, when we find the need for the same essence we just took as a result of the basic test (in the example it was Yellow Yarrow), it is because the symptom itself requires a direct infusion of that essence. Taking it in regard to the overall picture didn't do the trick.

Finding what essences are needed for a specific symptom is only half of the telegraphing procedure. It is equally important that you maintain that link while taking the essences. This moves the "essence" of the essences right through that linkup and into the symptom or specific area involved. The flower essence doesn't "get lost" this way. It moves right into the problem area, immediately locks into the electrical circuitry that is directly associated with this area, and reconnects and balances that circuitry. That's why it is not unusual to see and/or feel an immediate improvement in the symptom.

What I pass on to you here comes from my years of using the essences and the observations I've made as a practitioner of flower essences. This has to do with the relationship between what we are presently experiencing in our life and an accident. I have found that just as there is an underlying cause for why we are sick or feel under the weather, there is also a similar underlying issue attached to the injuries resulting from an accident. And often, the accident brings that issue to a head, and dealing with the individual injuries is an opportunity to recognize and release the issue and its energy. This energy gets released right through the injury itself. So don't be surprised (if you have been injured) if after doing the telegraph procedure you end up with flower essences that look suspiciously like a combination you might use to address the trauma of a rocky time in your marriage or a job change or fear of retirement.

I'll give you a rather dramatic example of this. We had friends visiting us a few years ago. While here they decided to help us clear a small road through our woods to the back property. The husband accidentally disturbed a nest of yellow jackets. They protested mightily and stung him three times. Now, for those of you who don't have such excitement in your life, getting stung by a yellow jacket is like getting hit at point-blank range with a poison arrow. By the time the husband quickly left the area and ran the five hundred feet to where I was at the house, his entire body was swelling, his eyes were nearly swollen shut, his lips were blue and swollen to about twice their normal size, and his overall coloring was bluish-white. Our closest hospital is a half-hour away and I didn't think he could survive the trip. Also, we did not have bee-sting antidote on hand. And I didn't think a couple of aspirins and encouraging words were going to help this fellow.

I got the flower essences and began testing. On the basic test he showed he needed essences that dealt with the shock of the trauma he was going through. No surprises. When I gave him those drops, nothing in his physical appearance changed. I then began telegraphing. I tested each sting separately and gave him the essences he needed for each before moving on to the next. All the essences were different, and that's when I noticed he was testing for essences that had no logical bearing on insect stings, serious or otherwise. (An additional moral to this story is to put aside judgment and logic at these times and give a person what they test as needing.) Also, after testing and giving him the needed essences for the first two stings, he showed no overall physical improvement. The only hopeful sign was that he wasn't getting worse. I tested the third sting. Again different essences. The minute he took these essences, all of his body symptoms reversed and visibly improved. We watched his coloring come back and the swelling recede. It took no more than fifteen minutes and all he was left with were three small, red welts. All along, I was not taking time to explain the definitions of the essences he was testing for. I just wrote them down. When we finally went over the definitions, it hit him that they were directly related to personal growth issues he had been going through — and not really wanting to face.

I am not saying that our friend got attacked by yellow jackets because of some personal growth issues he preferred to avoid. What I am saying is that in these situations there seems to be a relationship between the dynamic of the energy (usually emotional) surrounding a personal challenge or growth issue and the dynamic of a physical injury. The human system is very efficient and equally clever. The instant our friend was stung, his system registered the similarities between the dynamics of the sting and the dynamics of his personal issues and fused them appropriately to each sting. So I as the tester was no longer dealing with just a sting, I was dealing with a unit of fused energy. As we physically moved the stings through their process, the energy from the underlying issues moved in tandem with that physical process. The result was that emotional energy which had been building had surfaced and been released through the physical vehicle of yellow jacket stings.

In my experience with this phenomenon, the fusing of such units happens instantaneously and without warning, and why the individual system chooses to pair the specific dynamics it does (other than the issue of like attracting like) is part of what I call that amazing mystery, magic, and extraordinary brilliance of the human system. I do know that when I use the telegraph procedure to test someone who has a collection of different injuries, I find that ninety-nine times out of a hundred, these units have been formed and must be addressed in order to fully relieve the injury or efficiently move it through its healing cycle.

So how does all of this boil down to everyday practice? I'll give you examples on how to approach different situations. If you have a head cold and you are coughing and sneezing, give yourself the basic test and then telegraph test the coughing, then the sneezing, and then any other discernable symptom like a headache. The flu: Telegraph test the headache, the congestion, the nausea, the pain in the chest, the pain in the right leg, and the pain in the left leg. Asthma: Telegraph test the coughing, the breathing problem, and the congestion. Arthritis: If the joints of one hand are in pain, I would suggest that if you don't receive relief by testing the hand as a whole, test the joints separately. There may be a relationship among all the areas that won't be relieved until they are addressed separately. I know this sounds very tedious, but it may make the difference between getting or not getting the relief you need. Allergies: Telegraph test each symptom separately and each separate location of the symptom on the body. Poison ivy: You have it on the right wrist, left cheek, in back of the left knee, and on the top of your right foot. Telegraph test each location separately. As shown with the yellow jacket stings, treat accidents, injuries, and symptoms by addressing the location of each problem.

In short, treat overall conditions by addressing the individual symptoms or locations. Each symptom is serving some kind of purpose or it wouldn't be there. Now, you don't have to dissect yourself on the spot. Simply sit down and make a mental checklist of the obvious or what feels lousy. You may get the same essences for all the different locations or symptoms. If you do, take the essences again for each test.

By now you are probably saying, "Okay, okay, I get the idea!" But I'll warn you about something. In the beginning, this is a little harder to do than one might imagine, because basically we're used to thinking in terms of the whole rather than the collection of the parts. We say we have a cold or flu and have no conscious awareness of the various discomforts that comprise the illness. To keep from sounding like nit-pickers or hypochondriacs, we deal with such things as one unit. So the first few times we sit down to make this checklist or look at the bruises and scrapes we got when we fell, it takes a little bit of effort and focused attention to see, feel, and separate the situation into its parts. Once you make the checklist, take a couple of minutes to think about the symptoms you felt were unimportant, but are there. Then add them to the list too.

If you're not sure if the poison ivy or rash or whatever on the front of the left knee should be treated the same or separately as the poison ivy that is also on the side of the left knee, you can focus on the two areas and ask, "Are these two areas to be treated as one unit?" (Or with something like arthritis, ask, "Are the joints on my hand to be tested as one unit?") Do a kinesiology test and if you get a positive, test the essences for the two areas as a unit. If you get a negative, keep them separated.

Lastly. Here's a terrific telegraphing trick. If you are having difficulty linking with and/or holding your focus with a specific symptom or injury, just touch it. Even allow yourself to make it hurt *a little*. By doing this, you are "activating" that specific spot, and for a short period of time (about fifteen minutes), the entire body and mind automatically focus on that spot. Thus you have your link. To "deactivate" that spot in order to move on and test the next one, just lightly hit or touch the next spot. Your body and mind will shift focus immediately. The main thing to remember is that the touch must be enough to create some physical sensation. It can't be one of those feather-light, I-can't-feel-it touches.

Steps for Telegraph Testing

1. Do the basic essence test and take the needed essences. Make sure you are clear from the basic test before going on.

If you test for no essences, do the telegraph testing anyway. Not needing essences for the basic test but needing them for the more specific telegraph test is not unusual and demonstrates why telegraph testing is effective.

2. Make a checklist (mentally or, better yet, written) of all the various symptoms or injuries. Also separate them according to their different locations.

3. Link with your focus on each symptom or injury at each location, one at a time, and telegraph test. Make sure your focus is strong, clear, and that you maintain the link throughout the test. Touch the spot if necessary. Take the needed essences for the one symptom and find out how many days and how many times per day you are to take these essences. Also maintain your focus and link with the symptom or injury while taking the essences.

4. When all the symptoms/injuries have been treated, ask:
    Are all the symptoms/injuries now clear? (Test)
If negative, go through your checklist one by one asking:
    Is this symptom/injury clear? (Test)
Do another telegraph test for whatever tests negative. Then ask again if the symptoms/injuries are clear.

5. When you get a positive, ask:
    Am I clear generally? (Test)
If negative, do another basic essence test. This just means that there was a reaction during the telegraph testing, and a basic test is needed again for overall balancing. Take the essences needed and ask again if you are clear. This time, you'll get a positive. If by chance you don't, just do the basic test again.

6. When taking the essences for any of the symptoms/injuries for a prescribed period of time, focus your attention on each one while taking its essences.

HELPFUL HINTS FROM A SYMPATHETIC PRACTITIONER: As you've read, I haven't been sick very much during the past ten years. That, after all, is the point of using the flower essences. But I remember very well when I had that flu. The essences moved the two-week flu through its cycle and out of my system in less than a day. Three cheers for the result! However, getting the energy to sit up, even to look at all those little bottles, while I was in the midst of this flu was real tough. Working my fingers seemed akin to a ten-mile mountain hike. I think it's fair to say that one of the last things in the world we want to do when we're sick is flower essence testing. I clearly remember dragging myself through the testing and thinking, 'There's something to be said about taking those flu capsules.' Now that I've seen the results of my herculean efforts, it may still be a drag if I'm ever faced with a similar situation – but I'll have a stronger sense of purpose and this will help get me through it.

Here's my suggestion. If you don't have the energy to face telegraph testing while you're sick, concentrate on doing just the basic test. And don't even bother doing the dosage test for number of days and times per day. Do the basic test *every two hours* and take one drop of concentrate for each essence needed. Or put nine drops of each essence concentrate in a four-ounce glass of water and sip it during the next two hours as part of your liquid intake. But be sure to do the basic test every two hours. Your illness will be moving through its stages rapidly, and you will probably need different essences to support each new stage. If you don't need essences for one two-hour period, great, but test again at the start of the next two-hour period.

When you feel up to it, switch over and do the more precise telegraph testing in order to move through the final stages even more quickly.

Telegraphing: Serious Illness or Disease

Telegraphing is also useful when dealing with serious illness or disease. Cystic fibrosis, muscular dystrophy, multiple sclerosis, AIDS, cancer . . . In order to use the essences well in these circumstances, you must first know something about what the disease is and how it manifests. Then you need to apply that information to yourself and discern which aspects of the disease you are dealing with. If some of the symptoms are too subtle, simply make a list of the symptoms in question and do a kinesiology test for each, asking:

Does this symptom apply to me? (Test)

Once you have broken the disease into the various parts that apply to you, do the telegraph testing on each part. If you can physically locate on or in your body the specific symptom, focus your attention there as you do the testing. And maintain that focus as you take the essences.

If the symptom is too subtle or all-encompassing (such as a blood disorder), you may approach the focus necessary for telegraphing in two ways. One, you can use a written description of the symptom as the focal point. Make the description brief and concise — a few words or a couple of sentences. Then concentrate your attention and focus on this as you do the testing and take the essences. What this does is completely focus your mind and your brain on one thing to the exclusion of all else. In turn, the focus of your body is also on that one thing. This sets up the telegraph link. When you take the essences while maintaining this focus, they are telegraphed to the areas affected by the symptom upon which you are focused. Instead of using a physical pain or obvious physical sighting, as we did with the yellow jacket stings, you are using words.

Two: You can choose a visual symbol that for you embodies the symptom in relationship to your body. Again, this is very helpful if it is difficult to pinpoint the location of a symptom in the body. Instead of words, the one symbol stands for the symptom and its effect on the body. Whenever you wish to test this particular symptom, either picture the symbol in your mind or look at it drawn on paper, and maintain your focus on it throughout the testing and administering of the essences. It works exactly the same way as looking at the words in that your focus on the symbol excludes everything else but what is represented by the symbol. For both processes, the quality of focus has to be similar to the focus you would need if you were still trying to hear someone while standing in the middle of the New York Stock Exchange.

If all of this sounds familiar to you, it's probably because it is! Visualization therapy is used more and more these days in the treatment of serious illnesses, especially cancer. Physicians have found that treatment is much more effective if the patient visualizes what the treatment is supposed to be doing in the body. They give the patient all the clinical information that is needed and then let the patient go to work developing a visualization that embodies either symbolically or in realistic terms what is supposed to be happening to them. The visualization links the treatment right into the problem areas, which then enhances the effectiveness of the treatment. The relationship between the focused visualization and the physical movement of the treatment and its reaction on the body is not a chance thing. It is a discernable, viable relationship that is set up through the use of focus.

A word about the focus issue: In the beginning, achieving and maintaining this focus is going to be a little challenging. But developing focus is like developing muscle. If you work at it, the ability to focus strengthens. The body and mind learn what needs to happen in order to do this kind of focus. I'm not talking about some mystical-like paranormal achievement here. I'm literally talking about what you would need to do in order to fully hear someone who is speaking to you in the midst of chaos. We all can do this. Using the essences to their full potential requires that we develop this level of focus as a tool so that it can be called up anytime to be used quickly and efficiently.

Actually, before you get overwhelmed with the tedious tone of all of this, we are further ahead, on the whole, in our ability to focus than we are in muscle development! We are more a mental society and, for the most part, we already have the tools in place for the kind of focus I'm talking about. They just need to be sharpened. If you can read an interesting book for thirty minutes straight and be aware of nothing else but what you are reading, you know how to focus. There is nothing between you and the book. It's the same focus that is used when listening to someone in a chaotic atmosphere—only you have to work harder to achieve the focus that excludes everything but the person to whom you are listening.

When I describe focus in these terms, all I am doing is giving you an idea of what to shoot for when you sit down to test the flower essences. But because testing flower essences is different from reading a terrific book or listening in chaos, the focus that you already know is going to have to be applied to the flower essence testing and developed accordingly. It's a new situation. In a short period of time, you'll notice that your ability to focus will feel more agile, more in control, and more laser-beamed.

Steps for Telegraphing Serious Illness

1. Do the basic essence test. Take the needed essences and make sure you are clear. Make sure you are doing the testing during a time when you are not groggy (or at your least groggy time) from medication.

2. List the various symptoms that pertain to the illness.

3. Indicate which symptoms pertain to you. If you are unsure, test the questionable symptoms by asking:
Does this symptom apply to me? (Test)
If you intuitively feel there is a symptom you should address but the doctors aren't talking about this being a part of your disease, test if that symptom applies to you. If you get a positive, put it on the list. Remember, medicine doesn't know a lot about some of the diseases, and you may be getting an idea they haven't publicly (or privately) acknowledged yet.

4. Link with and telegraph test each symptom, one by one. Take the needed essences after each test and find out how many times a day and how many days/weeks/months you are to take these essences before moving on to the next test. You may wish to keep a record of the essences needed for each symptom. In time, they may create a pattern that could be useful for you to see and understand.

5. Test to see if the symptoms are clear by asking:
Am I clear regarding all the symptoms? (Test)
If negative, go through the list of symptoms one by one, asking:
Does this symptom need further testing? (Test)

If you get a positive, do another telegraph test for that symptom and take the essences that are needed. Then ask again if you are clear regarding the symptoms. Keep doing this until you get a positive.

6. Test to see if you are clear generally. Ask:

Am I now generally clear? (Test)

If negative, you then need to conclude this procedure by doing another basic test. There was a reaction during the telegraph testing, and you need to restore overall balance once more. Take the needed essences. Then ask again:

Am I now clear? (Test)

You'll get a positive, I'm sure. If you don't, do the basic test again until you are clear.

7. Do frequent follow-up testing of all the symptoms. Test after a prescribed dosage is completed in order to go on to the next step. Also, during periods when essences aren't being taken, check about once a week to see if any are needed by setting up for a telegraph test and going down the checklist of symptoms. If they test negative, you still don't need any for now. If they test positive, do the telegraph test for that symptom.

Telegraphing: Dealing with Serious Injuries

You're laid up in the hospital with, among other things, both arms in a cast and I'm suggesting you do extensive kinesiology with your fingers. You can cry "foul" and have a good laugh at my silliness. But I have a couple of ways around this little situation. It's as vital now to use the flower essences as ever. The healing process is enhanced in every way when the electrical system is connected, balanced, and strong. The trauma of an accident always blows or overloads the electrical system immediately. So it's imperative to get it rebalanced and maintain that balance throughout the entire healing process.

Of course it would be terrific if a friend or member of the family knew how to do surrogate testing and could take this chore completely off our shoulders at this time. If you were smart enough to help someone else learn how to use the essences, you've got your answer to the dilemma. Get that person by your side and working as soon as possible.

For the lone rangers who have no one willing to learn surrogate testing, now is the time to lean on intuition. You really have no choice. A key to getting strong intuitional insight is clarity. That is, tell yourself exactly what you want to know. Orchestrate yourself and keep it simple, as if you were setting up a question for kinesiology. This gives you internal order and clarity and creates the kind of clear environment needed for "hearing" intuition.

At the first quiet moment when you are able to deal with the essences, direct yourself to receive intuitively the essences you need by asking:

Which flower essences do I need generally?

This sets you up to do the basic test. Either allow the needed essences to just pop up in your mind or look at each bottle in the box and choose whichever essences stand out to you. If you can't do anything else but this simplified form of basic testing, that's fine. Take the essences and don't even bother doing the dosage testing. Assume that you are to take them three times a day—unless something to the contrary comes to mind. Also plan to do this testing once each day. If you can intuitively get the times per day and the number of days, that's great, but you don't have to push it. Have someone put nine drops of each essence in a four-ounce glass of water for you to sip at least three times throughout the day.

As soon as you are able to concentrate a little longer, add telegraph testing for your injuries. You may feel a little uneasy using intuition as your sole tool, especially when you have gotten used to kinesiology, but you have nothing to lose and everything to gain by trying. Let your gut instinct do the talking. Remember, if you are wrong, the body will cast off or reject the essence.

Steps for Telegraph Testing Serious Injuries

1. Do the basic flower essences test and take the needed essences. If you are incapacitated, you'll need someone to help you move essence bottles around, unscrew caps, and put the drops in water. So have an assistant on hand.

2. When you are ready for telegraph testing, make a checklist of your injuries – all of them, including the minor stuff you think is unimportant.

3. Link with and telegraph test each injury one by one. If necessary, touch each spot to "activate" it while you focus. (When using intuition, visually skim along the bottles for each injury, picking out whichever bottles attract you.) Take the needed essences for each injury while remaining focused on that injury. If you can't remain focused any longer, assume you're to take them three times a day. If possible, test or intuitively discern how many times a day and how many days the essences for each injury are to be taken.

4. When all the injuries have been treated, ask:
   Am I now clear regarding all the injuries?

If you test or discern negative, just go through the injury list one by one, asking:

Am I clear with this injury?

Whichever tests or feels negative, link with and do the telegraph testing again.

5. When all on the checklist tests or feels positive, ask:

Am I clear generally?

If you sense a negative on this, do the basic test again to make sure the entire electrical system is connected, balanced, and strong.

6. Do frequent follow-up testing. If you can't bother getting the number of days just yet, plan to do a telegraph test each day for all the injuries. If you can get the number of days and times per day, test each injury when the prescribed period of time ends. All the way through the recuperation and rehabilitation period, stay very close to the flower essences, testing frequently to make sure everything on the electrical level is in order. This entire period will move far more rapidly.

Now, you may feel that the idea of doing all this testing under such circumstances is nuts and that the possibility of doing accurate testing using intuition under these conditions is equally as nuts, but you will surprise yourself when you see how far a little bit of quiet, a little bit of determination, and a little bit of focus and order can get you. If you find yourself in this kind of crisis situation and you are experiencing all kinds of doubt and skepticism about the need to do this and your ability to pull it off, just try it once. If you set it up as I've suggested, you'll get the information you need. Once you take the essences, you'll sense or feel the difference they make, and that in itself will encourage you to continue the testing.

Telegraphing for Surgery

If you have not done so beforehand, begin using the essences and telegraph test whatever part of you is being scheduled for surgery as soon after diagnosis as possible. This will help you and the area slated for surgery to be fully prepared electrically. This is definitely not the time to be entering something half out of kilter. You will be focusing on either the specific organ in question or the area of the body where surgery is to take place — whichever applies best to the situation. And as with the other telegraphing procedures, you'll need to take the essences for the prescribed number of days, then retest for what is needed next, all the way up to the surgery.

Let me give you some examples: If you are having heart surgery, you should test the heart and the chest area where the incision is to be made. You don't have to be precise about the location of the incision, just the general area. If you are having heart and bypass surgery, test the valves or arteries involved, then the heart, and then the general incision area. If you are having a tumor removed, test the tumor itself, the area surrounding the tumor, and the area where the actual incision is to be made. If a wart is being removed, test the wart and the immediate surrounding area. If you are having an appendectomy, test the appendix, the immediate surrounding area, and the general incision area. In short, you'll need to address what the surgeon is aiming for and what he has to go through to get there.

HINT: You have the right to know what is going to happen to you. If you ask your doctor to explain what's involved in the surgery and what parts of your body will be affected, he'll tell you. Take notes and use what he says as the basis for your flower essence testing.

ANOTHER HINT: Normally the hospital will put you on a full fast prior to surgery. You can get around the fast by placing a drop of each needed essence concentrate, one drop at a time, on your forehead and lightly rubbing it into the skin. Or you can place one drop of each needed essence concentrate on your lips. The drop will slowly enter the mouth and gradually mix with the saliva. Do whichever process you feel comfortable with, and if you aren't sure, just test to see which process is best for you at that time. This way you can keep the essence process going right up to surgery.

There is an additional telegraphing test you'll want to do as part of the preparation. When you have completed testing the areas/organs in question, focus back on yourself as if you were going to do a basic test, think of the surgery facing you, and ask:

Do I need any essences to help prepare me for this surgery?
(Test)

If positive, test the essences while keeping your mind on the surgical situation that faces you. While maintaining this focus, take whatever essences test positive. What you are looking at here is the effect the coming surgery has on you generally—what it is for you to face this situation. This is a form of telegraphing in which the link isn't to a specific body area but rather to the surgery as an upcoming and inevitable event, and its effect on you overall. In short, how does the trauma of facing surgery throw you, disconnect you electrically? If you need no essences, you are doing fine with accepting and dealing with the idea of going through surgery. This doesn't mean you're not frightened or concerned. It just means that those feelings are not overpowering you electrically.

If you do need essences, they tell us not only what part of the surgery troubles you most but also that whenever you spend time thinking, talking, and worrying about the surgery you will probably unbalance or disconnect electrically and need these essences. So if in the first telegraph test you thought about the surgery and found out, for example, that you needed Broccoli Essence just one time rather than for several days or every day up to the surgery, this means you will also most likely need Broccoli Essence one time after each subsequent worry session. You can assume this and just take a drop of Broccoli Essence after you've caught yourself worrying, talking, and thinking. Or, after these moments, concentrate on yourself for a couple of seconds and ask, "Do I need Broccoli Essence now?" Take a drop if you do. If you are especially good at hiding things from yourself and really aren't consciously aware of the times you are worrying about the surgery, test yourself for Broccoli Essence a couple of times a day on general principle.

So with the issue of surgery, you'll need to keep two things in mind: 1) the preparation of the area/organ to be operated on and 2) the effect facing surgery is having on you overall. If you find that you are having to do testing on almost a daily basis—that is, the area/organ test is using essences for one or two days only and then you are testing for new essences—you can combine tests #1 and #2 as a matter of course. If, however, test #1 calls for one series of essences to be taken every day up to the surgery, you'll need to pay frequent attention to test #2 on its own.

One last thing: As with illness and injury, there is an underlying reason why you are now faced with a surgical situation. The essences that come up will identify this for you. Usually the essences for the core issue pop up during the week prior to surgery. So pay attention to what essences come up. Complete recuperation after surgery will rest in part on your addressing this core issue and making the appropriate changes in your life.

Telegraph Testing Steps for Surgery Preparation

1. Do the basic essence test. Take the essences needed. Test to make sure you are clear before going on.

2. Make a mental or written checklist of the organs and/or areas involved in surgery. (If you write it down, you won't have to rethink this every time you test.) If you are questioning whether an area should be treated as one unit or broken down into several smaller areas or parts, focus on the area and ask:

Is this to be treated as one unit? (Test)

If negative, list the parts as you understand them. [You don't have to take Anatomy 101 for this. Just let what you know and what comes to mind be your guide. *Or*, if you want more precision, you can purchase at just about any bookstore an anatomy coloring book which shows the human body in a very simple, easy-to-understand way. (For information, see *Bibliography and Resources*.) Turn to the area you're interested in and use their pictures as your guide. Go through the list of parts asking, "Am I to test this?" What tests positive goes on your checklist.]

3. Link with and telegraph test everything on your checklist, one by one, taking the needed essences for each before going on to the next test. Remember to keep your focus on the area or organ during both the test and while taking the drops of essences.

4. When all the telegraph testing is complete, ask:

Are all the specific areas now clear? (Test)

If negative, go back through the list one by one, asking:

Is this area/organ clear? (Test)

Do a telegraph test for whatever tests negative and take the essences needed. Then ask again if the specific areas are clear. When all test positive, move on to the next step.

5. Return your focus to yourself in general, as if you were preparing for a basic test. Think of the surgery that faces you. When that is clearly in your mind (take a half-minute to fully focus your attention on the surgery), ask:

Do I need any essences in order to help prepare me for this surgery? (Test)

If positive, test the essences while remaining focused on the surgery and maintain that focus as you take the drops. Also maintain the focus while you check for how many days and how often each day you are to take these essences. (Whenever you take them, it is important that you focus on the surgery in order to properly telegraph the essences.) If you test that you need to take the essences only one time, then it will be safe to assume you may need a drop after worrying, thinking, or talking about the surgery and that these essences should be checked as mentioned previously.

6. Return your focus to yourself generally for a final basic test and ask:

Am I now clear? (Test)

If negative, do the basic essence test again. Take the needed essences and ask once more if you are clear. Do this until you test positive to the question.

7. Do follow-up testing for each area or organ as its prescribed essence period ends.

After Surgery

Now, you've come through the surgery and have before you the recovery and rehabilitation period. Approach the essences exactly as you would if you were recovering from an accident. Use the steps I listed for *Serious Injury Or Accident*. Your checklist will be the same as what you used prior to surgery plus anything that might have become unexpectedly involved during surgery. You will not need to do the telegraph test now for how the impending surgery was affecting you (Step 5). As soon as possible after surgery, do a basic test for yourself and do the follow-up when this essence period ends. When you are able to concentrate more, add the telegraph testing to the basic test. As mentioned in the section *Serious Injury or Accident*, you may not be able to or feel up to using your fingers. Don't hesitate to use intuition until you have enough strength to switch to the fingers. Continue the regular testing during the entire period of recovery and rehabilitation. If it takes a year, stay close to the essences throughout that entire year. The pattern you will see now in the essences will be related to not only the physical and emotional rehabilitation process regarding the surgery itself but also to the stabilizing and balancing needed as you face the underlying cause(s) of the surgery in the first place.

A helpful word about long-term testing: On the surface it sounds exhausting and tedious, I know. But once you settle into the flower essence pattern that you need, it won't be unusual for you to find that you'll be on a specific collection of essences for weeks or even months at a time. This is true for any of the testing. In an emergency, we may be talking about the need to test hourly, daily, or every few days. But this is in response to the crisis and is temporary. Once you are over the crisis, the essence patterns lengthen and even out. I'm emphasizing the need for diligence because it is so important that you not go through one series of essences and then let it drop right there without checking to see if there is a follow-up series. If you miss the follow-up, you can lose a lot of the benefits from the initial series. Healing and change have a building-block process. But in my desire to emphasize the need for diligence, I may be sounding as if you will be testing flower essences every waking hour. This simply isn't so.

As you have probably figured out, I use flower essences extensively in my own life. However, they are so integrated into my life that I am barely aware of any time it takes for me to test and use them. It's like brushing my teeth — I just do it, but I don't walk around feeling burdened by it. What I think you need to do to gain some confidence about how gracefully and gently the flower essences move through your life is to learn to use them in a general way and not wait for a crisis that might require more frequent use. You'll see how gracefully they pattern out and the lengthy periods of time when absolutely no flower essences are needed. Then when an emergency arises, you'll know full well that the additional focus on the essences is needed but temporary.

Telegraphing Structural Misalignments

This is a little trick I've learned over the years because my friendly neighborhood chiropractor is an hour's drive away, and I wasn't about to go rushing off every time I felt misaligned. By "misaligned" I mean something like a vertebra that is not seated properly along the spinal column, or anything in the rest of the skeletal system that has been knocked, pulled, banged, or emoted out of its correct alignment. If as a matter of good health rather than because of an accident you have gone to a chiropractor, you probably noted that there was a pattern of adjustments. You have a tendency to have the same or related adjustments repeated each time, and if you think about it, you also have a tendency to feel the same pains. The pains are the result of the misalignments, and it is usually the case that a person will wait until that pain reaches a particular level of discomfort before taking the time to see the chiropractor.

In order to use the flower essences in this process, you must be willing to allow yourself to feel the pain or the discomfort at the outset. This is a matter of sensitizing yourself. It's also easier said than done. We are very practiced at ignoring or not registering pain or physical change until it reaches the level where the discomfort is intolerable, and all of the related muscles have now become "locked" into stretches and scrunches that accommodate this misalignment. For this flower essence process, we have to teach ourselves to recognize and pair the early warning signs with the misalignment so that we'll know, for example, that as we're walking along and feel our left leg to be "shorter" than the right, this means the pelvis is misaligned on the left.

157

Asking the chiropractor questions about what he is adjusting and what might be an early warning sign that this adjustment is needed, plus learning to be more consciously aware of what your body signals are saying to you, provide a good approach to sensitizing yourself. He can give you an idea of what to look for in the early stages of a misalignment. Then it's up to you to pay attention.

The reason why I am saying all of this is because it is possible to realign the body structurally if we catch the problem within the first 72 hours of misalignment. Up to 72 hours, the misalignment isn't "locked" into position. After this period of time, the muscles and even your body movement have altered to accommodate this new "alignment," making it impossible to use something as subtle as flower essences to achieve correction.

So, let's get down to practicality here. You have a tendency for a cervical vertebra to misalign. You have learned that when you feel a certain ache in the neck, that's the indication that the cervical vertebra is out again. You've taught yourself to feel that ache right at the outset. You're bopping along in life feeling just great when all of a sudden you feel the subtle twinges of that pain in the neck. As soon as possible, test yourself for essences.

Steps for Testing Structural Misalignments

1. Do the basic flower essence test first, taking the needed essences and checking for the number of days and times per day you are to take these essences. Make sure you are clear generally before going on.

2. Do a telegraph test using the pain as your focus. This puts you right into the area of the misalignment. Test and take the needed essences while remaining focused on the pain. Also test

for number of days and times per day you are to take the essences. If you know precisely what is out of alignment and where it's located, you can also telegraph test this. Focusing on the actual structural misalignment is a bit tougher than focusing on the pain. I have found that either focus gets results.

3. Check to make sure you are clear regarding the telegraph testing. Ask:

Am I clear regarding this alignment problem? (Test)

If the response is negative, keep telegraph testing the area, taking the essences, and checking to see if it's clear until you get a positive.

4. Check yourself generally to make sure you are clear. Ask:

Am I clear generally? (Test)

If negative, do the basic test again. Take the needed essences and test for clearing again. Do this until you get a positive response to the question.

I generally get results within twenty minutes of taking the essences. First the pain subsides, and then any structural discomfort leaves. If I did the test because as I was walking, one leg felt shorter than the other, that sensation was gone after the essence testing. I make sure I do all the follow-up testing in order to maintain the balance needed for the body to fully realign.

Now, the flower essences are not in the body acting as bulldozers pushing bones around. What has happened is that something has caused an electrical disconnection or imbalance which, rather than weakening an organ, gland, or muscle, has instead registered structurally. So by immediately addressing the underlying cause, the reason for the structural misalignment is eliminated. Instantaneously, the body components—the muscular, skeletal, nervous, and electrical systems—will work to restore the previous alignment.

There's an important bit of information the essences give you in this process. If you have a tendency to "throw out" your cervical vertebrae, the essences give you feedback that lets you know what in your life situation affects your neck on a regular basis. So instead of waiting for the neck to start hurting, you can work either to eliminate the situation or alter the pattern of your reaction, thus resolving the neck problem altogether.

One more thing. There is a reverse angle to this process. That is, you're bopping through life just fine and on general principle or because you notice you're feeling a little off, you sit down to do a basic essences test. Much to your surprise you test a need for fourteen flower essences. That's about twelve more than you usually test for. Whenever you discover the need for a bunch of essences—I'd say over ten, but if six seems unusually high to you, then consider six to be a bunch—you may be structurally misaligned and need to see a chiropractor. This kind of essence result usually means you're "out," you've been that way for awhile, and your electrical system (among other things) is short-circuiting and overloading all over the place. This isn't a sure-thing situation, so before you reach for a phone book to find a chiropractor, bring your focus to yourself generally and ask:

Do I need to see a chiropractor? (Test)

Or:

Am I structurally misaligned? (Test)

A positive for either question means you do need to reach for the phone book. Take the flower essences you have tested for and take them as prescribed, plus do follow-up testing, if necessary, until you have your appointment. This will stabilize you electrically even though, by this time, they won't help the structural problem. Then after seeing the chiropractor, test the essences again and take them for the prescribed period of time.

Surrogate Telegraph Testing

If you are surrogate testing for someone who needs telegraph testing, here's how you set it up. Link with the person exactly as described in Chapter 7 on *Surrogate Testing*. Go through all the various steps, making sure that you clear yourself first by doing the basic test before doing any testing on the person. When it's time to telegraph test, it is better if the person you are testing focuses on the specific areas. They create the link. So if someone has had heart surgery and you are getting ready to telegraph test the heart, just ask them to focus on their heart (or heart area) and hold that focus while you do the testing with the bottles. Give them a minute to settle their focus on the specific area. If they have pain in the area, tell them to focus on the pain. That's usually an easy focus for them. And if your testing is more on the slow side, periodically (and softly) remind them to maintain focus on the area being tested. These reminders help direct their focus and keep their mind from wandering. When you give them the essences, they are still to have the specific area in mind.

For surrogate testing people who cannot do the focus or telegraph link themselves — infants and children, comatose people, folks who are simply too weak or too groggy — you as the tester need to take over this function. Set yourself up and link with these people as with any surrogate testing situation. Do the basic essence test and give them the essences. If they are unable to take the essences, for adults and children you can place one drop of each concentrate on the lips (dilute the drop in a little bit of water if they object to the brandy taste), and for infants up to three months old, you can put a drop of each concentrate on the forehead. Although adults and children older than three months can also have the drops administered on their foreheads, the flower essences move more efficiently and effectively into their nervous system if they are taken orally. Prior to three months of age, the nervous system is equally sensitive to skin application as it is to oral administration. I recommend that for anyone older than three months, the essences be given orally unless they're in an impossible situation such as a strict fast before surgery.

When it's time to telegraph test, you focus your attention on the area you wish to test. Make sure your focus is on the area or organ in their body and *not in yours*. You can do this in several ways:

1. If what you are testing is visible, simply "rest" your attention/focus visually right on it. In other words, look at it, make the connection, and mentally hold that connection while you do the test and the administering of the drops. Or you can touch the area to physically "activate" it. Then link your focus into the area and remember to maintain that focus while you are administering the drops. Touching the area again just before giving the drops assures that the spot is still activated.

2. If it is not a surface area, you can look at the general area with the intent of linking with the area or organ beneath the surface, make the connection mentally, and hold that connection during the test and administering of the drops.

3. Say (aloud or to yourself), "I wish to be linked to Mary's heart for testing." Your focus on that intent creates the link. Sense the link having been established (sometimes you can "feel" that link occurring) and mentally hold it while you test and administer the essences.

4. Visualize a thin line connecting you to the area you wish to test. This will serve to actually create the link. Maintain the sense of that visualization as you do the testing and administering of the drops.

Whatever method you use, you can verify that you are linked by asking (for example):

Am I linked to Mary's heart? (Test)

If negative, *relax*, eliminate anything that might be distracting you, and attempt the link again.

This surrogate-linking business is really not difficult to do. It does take some quiet and a bit of focus. But if you've been doing surrogate testing for others, you'll find that this situation won't be hard to pull off.

Once one telegraph test is completed, disconnect your link with that area/organ (remove your focus or visualization) and prepare to link with the next area or organ for the next test. Just keep verifying each link, maintain a gentle mental focus on that link, and trust your testing.

TESTING YOUR FAMILY OR GROUP

If you are introducing flower essences into your life and you live in a family or close-knit home group, it would be helpful to extend flower essences to the other members. By definition, an immediate family or group has such a close level of interaction that when one of its members moves through change or faces stress and trauma, some or all of the others also react or respond. Two things can happen: 1) You, for example, can be going through a process that is threatening to someone close — either the fact that *you* are the one going through this, or the event or cause of the process itself can be threatening to them. 2) In a conscious or unconscious sympathetic gesture, the people around you can be absorbing the stress and trauma you are going through.

This latter situation can pop up with anyone in a family or close-knit group. But it is especially prevalent with children. Children often act as the emotional sponge of a family, and even when they are not being told about problems or changes, they pick right up on them. Their electrical systems are especially vulnerable as well as sensitive to these things. As a flower essence practitioner, I will do three things when children are a part of the picture: 1) If the parent is in process and being tested, I will automatically check the children as well to find out what, if anything, the children are absorbing that might be throwing them off balance. 2) If I am testing a child who is ill or showing changes in behavior patterns, and that child's test results indicate something beyond normal childhood process, I'll check the parents for essences. Generally, I'll find that the source of the situation lies with the parents. 3) If, after testing a child, I have any questions about whether or not the underlying causes for needing essences are child-based or adult-based, I'll check the adults just to be sure.

I can't stress enough how sponge-like children are. I know that if you are a parent, you are particularly aware of their sensitivity to what's going on around them. But working with the essences in these situations has made me far more aware of not only their sensitivity but also what they will absorb and how often they are knocked off kilter — especially when we adults are absolutely *sure* that we are successfully insulating the children from a particular situation. From my experience, I would say that it is safe to assume that children are being insulated from nothing. I would check them for essences on general principle anytime another member of the family or the family as a unit is involved in process or change.

Here's the most amazing thing about this issue with children. It is not unusual for me to test a child, look at the results and suspect it to be adult-based, confirm my suspicions by testing the parents, give *them* the needed essences, and turn right around and retest the child, only to find that the child no longer needs the essences. By treating and stabilizing the parents, the child's system automatically stabilized. When working with children, you can't assume that this phenomenon will occur every time adults are involved in the picture, but it can happen up to fifty percent of the time.

Children are especially vulnerable during times of major change within the family unit, like the birth of a baby or a family move, and during long-term serious illness of a family member. These types of situations are especially stressful and tend to draw our attention away from the child in order to focus on the major situation. I worked with a seriously ill (cystic fibrosis) infant who had a three-year-old brother. Everyone of course was focused on the infant's situation. When I tested the three-year-old, however, I got a full readout of the trauma everyone around the infant was experiencing, plus some of the infant's trauma as well. The older, healthy child was "on the sidelines" absorbing everything. He needed to be supported by the essences, but more importantly, the parents needed to take the time to recognize and address their own personal trauma and do something about it (use the essences, for example) before the pressure could be released from the shoulders of the healthy child.

In short, in order to maintain balance within a family or group unit, especially with the children, while change is occurring, pay attention to the essence needs not only of the children but of the adults—all of the adults. It is possible that the primary member going through the process may not need any essences at all—that person may be doing just fine with the situation. But one or more members surrounding that person may be threatened to pieces by the situation and blowing all kinds of circuits. The children will absorb from and become systemically unbalanced from the surrounding members, and the balance being maintained by the primary member will not stop the child's imbalance from occurring.

Children also act as the family barometer. Let's say you feel that life is going along smoothly right now. But suddenly your child either gets sick or changes normal behavior patterns. By "normal" I mean the established patterns of behavior, whether they change from one pattern to a better one or one pattern to a less pleasant one. This change could mean that something is happening in the family that no one else is willing to recognize or, if recognized, the family or member is unwilling to deal with it. Consequently, on the surface, everything appears to be fine, but the child has picked up on and responded to the hidden situation. Test the child for essences and administer them as prescribed. But it will be important to test everyone else whether or not the situation has been identified. Most likely what will happen is that one or more members will test for the peeling process. In order to hide the situation, they've layered it. And the child didn't pay any attention to all that sophisticated adult footwork.

Testing children during this kind of family situation tends to be quite simple. While you may have to do the peeling process or telegraph test adults, children will most likely only need a basic essence test to restore full balance and connection. You can check to make sure—which I completely recommend—by telegraph testing as the child thinks of the particular situation involved or, if the child is too young, by your taking the role of creating the link by focusing on the issue for the child and then telegraph testing. Do this exactly as described in the *Surrogate Telegraph Testing* section in this chapter. As I have said, you will most often find that the child will only need the basic test. This means that he is reacting to the issue as an overall situation that is encompassing his life in general, rather than breaking the issue down into specific areas of his life.

It may sound a bit overwhelming to be the person with the flower essences in a group or family during change or crisis. One thing I suggest is that if the other members are open to flower essences being included in their lives, urge them to learn to use the essences themselves. Then in these larger group situations, each person can take care of himself while you help the children. But human nature being what it is, don't be surprised if you get designated the "family practitioner" and they turn to you for testing during their time of need.

So, you have a situation and suspect that all five members of the family need to be checked for flower essences. To encourage you to put out the effort to test them, consider that it will be much less stressful and far more efficient for them to move through the situation as a balanced, fully functioning group unit than to have everyone trying to figure things out and acting while being blown, off balance, and out of kilter. It's sort of like trying to fly a plane with one wing missing. No matter how much you try, you probably won't get off the ground, and even though you could taxi to your destination, that's not the point of an airplane, and it certainly isn't very efficient.

To test this group, set yourself up in a quiet part of the house and really function as the practitioner. Have each person come to you individually and surrogate test them as you would for any one-on-one situation. *Be sure to test and clear yourself first.* And forget that four others are outside waiting. Keep a record of what they need, how many days they need it, and how often per day they should take it. Do the basic test first, then telegraph test the effect the specific situation is having on them. If they have any physical complaints—pain, headache, a new injury, restlessness, etc.—telegraph test these as well. They are most likely related to the situation. Tell the person which essences they need and make sure they have an idea of what those essences mean.

If the essences are to be taken for more than a couple of days, make a solution bottle. *Be sure to tape the person's name on the bottle.* Dropper bottles all look alike, any combination of flower essences smells alike, and people have the habit of leaving their bottles around. You get five people doing this and the situation gets completely out of control, fast. No one knows who belongs to which bottle. It would also be very helpful if you included on the taped-bottle information the number of days the solution is to be taken, times per day, and the date the solution bottle was made. If a person has to take a solution for eighteen days, it's hard to calculate when the period of days is over unless you know when it began. Or, you can just do the calculation for them and put the completion date for that solution on the label.

As the practitioner, it's important for you to keep a record of all of this information, including the specific essences they each need. It's a safe bet that two out of the five people are going to misplace their bottles, and the other three will forget some or all of what you've told them. Also, you'll need to coordinate the follow-up, and the record is what keeps you on top of this. Just figure out when each person's dosage ends, and write the end date either beside their name or as part of their personal record, or in a sequential list that has all the dates for the next test with the person's name written beside each date. The key to success here—plus the key to maintaining sanity—is to do whatever you must do to easily organize the flower essences testing. Once you do this, you'll see that it will be an easy issue to keep current with everyone's follow-up testing. Continue the follow-up throughout the entire situation, and you'll know everyone is through it when, as a result of their follow-up testing, they test clear in both the basic test and the telegraph test.

REMINDER: If you feel hungry after this kind of long testing session, you've depleted your body's protein and need to eat something high in protein. Do this immediately after the testing session.

There's a different kind of follow-up I'd like to suggest that you do, as well. After it's all over and everyone is through their part of the situation, or nearly through, sit back and look at what happened. Think of the issue and review how you as individuals and as a group responded and moved through it. Think of this in light of how all of you have moved through similar times before without using the essences. To take it further, look at the strengths and weaknesses that showed up within the group and within each individual during *this* time. The flower essences give excellent feedback for discovering patterns and pitfalls, and they can help strengthen your family as a functioning unit. One person learns how their reaction, while not necessarily unbalancing them, may intensify another's reaction to the same thing, causing them to unbalance.

Such a review and discussion would also serve to point out and help make everyone conscious of the difference the essences made. The next time around, everyone has a clearer idea of what the essences are doing and how they benefit by them, and they will have more of a desire to assist and cooperate with you as the flower essence practitioner. It's that old thing—that if people know what they are doing, why they are doing it, and recognize its validity, they feel purpose and are able to respond better.

Up to this point I've concentrated on the family or group within the context of home. There is the "family" or close-knit group within the context of work that can be considered, as well. This takes a combination of guts, sensitivity, and conviction on your part, and a little openness to something new on the others' part. I know it's one thing to be considered a little daffy by your family but quite another thing to be considered daffy in the workplace.

If you are working in a small business or in a small unit within a large business, and the quality of your work as a unit depends on the ability to work closely with one another, you might consider discussing the flower essences with these people. Now, I think it is good to wait until you have enough experience with the essences to explain them from the point of personal experience.

Also, think about what you are going to say before you say it. If you have a tendency to describe flower essences in esoteric, spaced-out language, think of a "straight" way to word it. I find that people feel much more comfortable hearing about new things if they don't sound like something that just landed from Mars. I make it a point to say what I want about these things in the language that is most comfortable for the person to whom I am speaking.

I also feel that it is important not to try to push flower essences if you have broached the subject and no one seems interested. There are issues of personal timing, appropriateness, and manipulation to consider here. So I recommend moving gently and with sensitivity to the reactions of others. (This also applies to someone in the family or home group who does not want to use flower essences.)

Close-knit work groups are a natural for incorporating flower essences, especially during times when everyone is working together in a stressful situation. Again, if you have an opportunity to respond to and move through a situation with all cylinders fully functioning, why choose to do it with anything less?

One way to gently incorporate the essences is to have a set available at work and offer to test someone who is not feeling well. Always explain what the essences are and what they do, and if the person gives you the okay, test them privately as you would anyone, doing the basic test first and any further testing, if necessary. The difference they feel from the essences will speak louder and more convincingly than anything we could possibly say about them. This always breaks the ice, not only for the person you've tested but also for the others when they hear from that person what happened.

Usually what will occur is that the others will begin to approach you, especially when they are not feeling well. In short, what you are doing is letting the others incorporate the essences into the office situation, rather than you trying to push the essences into that environment. It's my belief that this is not only the better approach but an appropriate approach, as well. Once they become at ease and a bit familiar with the essences, you might suggest that you as a group find out if essences are needed during a specific stressful time.

WITH THERAPEUTIC PROCESSES

I've mentioned before that flower essences are quite helpful while we are involved in a therapeutic process, whether it be emotional counseling or physical therapy. The goal of both is change. It seems to be human nature that when change is involved, we tend to dig in our heels and resist mightily, hoping above all else to hang on to what is familiar. Yet here we are putting ourselves in a therapeutic situation because we want to change. A bit of a conflict of interest arises here—a push/pull situation where on one hand we know we must change and we seek help to accomplish this, while on the other hand we dig in and resist because the idea of letting go of the familiar is so frightening. This friction is one of the issues flower essences can address. They won't eradicate the friction or the fears that arise from that friction, but they will make sure you are supported and stabilized while you deal with them.

A minor detour for a few general thoughts about fear. I put them here because physical and emotional therapeutic processes tend to both deal head on with fear as a block to change and, at the same time, do everything possible to stir us up so that we can experience more fear than we ever thought possible.

I've learned that there are two more things besides taxes and death that are inevitable. They are change and fear. The only way to avoid them is to clamp ourselves down so much that we become completely stagnant, changeless, and therefore have nothing to fear. If one considers that life is a never-ending process of evolution, then, I feel, it is reasonable to say that real death is existence without change. So if one chooses life, one must accept change — constantly. And along with change comes fear. This all may sound simplistic, but I am continually astonished at how many people I meet who don't realize that change and fear are simply two givens in their life and are not something to be sidestepped or avoided. They put a great deal of energy and effort into avoiding change because they can't seem to get beyond their fears about changing.

It's not that I am suggesting that there is no reason to fear change. I don't think that would be healthy. A good, balanced dose of fear fosters caution and common sense when we are faced with something new, and it keeps us from flying into the sun. What I am saying is that fear, along with change, is a given.

People are often astonished when I say to them that I experience fear often — constantly. I choose to live a life of constant change and exploration of the new. But I'm not stupid. I don't jump off the edge into the unknown without experiencing fear — sometimes a lot of fear. People perceive me to be a strong individual. And I am. *Very* strong. But they are shocked when I talk openly about my fears because they equate strength of character with fearlessness. What makes me strong is that I've figured out that change and fear are unavoidable, so I had better devise a workable system or two or three for getting through them. I treat change and fear as positive life components to be figured out and used well. I know how to move to the edge of the unknown and use fear to my advantage, in fact, as a tool to help keep me from being reckless. My goal in life is to discover as much as I possibly can about what life really is without self-destructing. So I've looked at how I approach and accomplish change and have devised frameworks that enhance the positive and avoid or control the weak aspects of my patterns. And I've looked at fear and devised systems that make it work *for* me and not against me. The point I try to make about fear is that we really don't eradicate it from our lives — it either rules us or we figure out how to use it to our best advantage.

So how did I do this? I can hear you asking that. It helped to be in a situation in my childhood — starting from age twelve when I became a "throw-away child" — where my physical survival depended on my ability to overcome the enormous fears I had about the situation. The fear of starving to death overrode all the fears I had about dealing with the adult society around me so that I could get up, get a job, and not starve to death. One major fear won out and overrode other critical but not-quite-so-major fears. So I learned early on that fears are blocks that can be, and at times must be, overridden.

Of course this is a good lesson and one that I find a whole bunch of people haven't picked up, even by the time they become forty. But then they didn't have the advantage of my early disadvantage! If you look at the dynamics of what I have described, you'll see that all I did in the early years was treat fear like wooden blocks to be moved around and repositioned in a way that would allow me to move forward. I didn't alter the fear itself, I just repositioned it.

As I got older, I began to see that fear is a dynamic that is both negative and positive, depending on how you look at it and how you wish to deal with it. I found that with all fear I've experienced, there are two sides—one side being fear as a block, the other side being fear as a tool. So rather than moving wooden blocks around, I began to look at my fear as I experienced it (rather than as one huge, all-encompassing collection called "fear") and worked to discover the aspect of it as a tool. In the process, I discovered fear to be intelligent, a valid early-warning system, a link to my higher self trying to get my conscious, sometimes stubborn self to catch on that what I am about to do is not really what I should be doing. In short, I found that fear plays right into gut instinct, and, at times, it is the dynamic that makes my gut react strongly and accurately to something. I found that fear is like a built-in wise Jewish mother who keeps constant vigilance over my safety and well-being.

Once I got to this point, I had a friend and a partner rather than an interfering force that needed to be moved out of my way before it rendered me immobile. I still experience fear—often. But it's taken on a different perspective and become part of my personal process of change. And this is something that I feel is supposed to occur. We start out experiencing them side by side. Fear and change. Change and fear. All I did was to take the hint and keep them together, and make them into a supportive team.

So how in the world do flower essences play into what I'm saying? Much of my development went on prior to ten years ago when I began using the essences. Since then, they have been responsible for the fine-tuning I've done in this area. Mind you now, I'm not suggesting I have hit some pinnacle of full mastery over change and fear. This growth process, like everything else, keeps changing! But the flower essences gave me input regarding how I change and deal with fear that I could not perceive or figure out in the previous years. The input was subtle, as I've said, fine-tuning in nature. And while using the essences as I moved through change, I was able to far more clearly see how my fears interweave and manifest throughout the process. They gave me specific and precise input, and this has allowed me to develop change and fear frameworks that allow me more agility and flexibility. Had I had the benefit of the flower essences early on, I don't believe I would have had to work nearly as hard at figuring out what I was really doing during times of change and fear. I would have had that precise input I speak of, and I don't think I would have felt I was shooting arrows into space quite so often.

I don't regret my past experiences nor my process for getting through them, painful and sometimes clunky though some were, but I don't see why we shouldn't "do it" better and more gracefully if given the chance. I don't think there's some kind of cosmic regulation that states that for certain life experiences we all are required to always experience the same process and its corresponding pain. In short, using flower essences facilitates this whole forward movement we're involved in — giving it levels of smoothness and grace and precision.

Essences do more than give you input. They stabilize fears as well. This is important when we're either over our heads or facing fear in new ways and have no concept for how to deal with it. If we're in a therapeutic situation, this is exactly how we feel! Now, there is a real difference between stabilized fear and electrically-shorted, runaway fear. The latter is exactly as it sounds, and we've all felt it. It's a powerful, out-of-control fear that feels to us impossible to deal with because the fear is in the driver's seat. In short, we are bullied by our own fear. It renders us weak and gives us the feeling that about all we can do is go to bed, curl up under the covers, and hope the whole thing—the fear and the situation causing the fear—will take care of itself and go away on its own. It is a safe bet that when we experience these feelings, that fear has shot beyond our perimeter of balance and we have overloaded or shorted electrically.

Stabilized fear allows us to maintain control. The fear is still there but we have the feeling from deep inside ourselves that we can look this fear, and the situation that is causing it, right square in the eye and do something constructive to resolve it. *We* remain in the driver's seat. Or, another way to say it is that we own the fear, it doesn't own us. Maintaining electrical balance literally gives us the internal support we need, resulting in that feeling of facing stabilized fear.

Back to therapeutic situations: If you are in counseling, test yourself for flower essences prior to and after each session. The test prior to the session makes sure that any apprehensions you might feel haven't blown or overloaded you and that when you walk in there, all circuits are connected and fully functioning. You are supported, and when fears rise to the surface during the session, you will experience them as supported fears. (On a more practical level, you get more for your money out of the therapy hour if you're not electrically bouncing off the walls and dealing with the resulting out-of-control feeling.) The test after the session reconnects and balances anything that has short-circuited or overloaded during the session and assists with the support you need in order to integrate what has occurred. It is important to this integration process that any follow-up testing be done until the next therapy session. Then start the process over, testing just prior to the session and again after, being sure to continue any follow-up that might arise from that new session. Treat the time just prior to the session, the session, and the period after the session and up to the next one as one unit.

For each test you will need to do basic testing and, most likely, telegraph testing. Prior to the session, the focus of the telegraph testing is that session facing you as a general process that might be causing you apprehension. (Similar to testing the effects pending surgery is having.) You don't have to try to figure out what might happen — or what you don't want to happen. Keep the focus general. Do this by simply visualizing yourself sitting in the office or room with your therapist. After the session, focus in a general way on what has just occurred (recreating a general experience the session gave you) or on something specific that especially sticks out in your mind. Let your intuition be your guide. You don't have to do this testing in the outer office before putting on your coat to go home. When you get home is soon enough. It should be done within an hour or two after the session. The same is true for the test prior to the session.

A little about physical therapies: By this I mean any physical therapy we must take after surgery or an accident that is for the purpose of restoring movement, plus the therapies beyond the usual medical setting such as the Alexander Technique, Feldenkrais, therapeutic touch or therapeutic massage. The general, overall theory here is that by teaching the body to move in different ways or affecting the movement of the body for the purpose of change, one is creating simultaneous movement of the individual on all other levels. The reverse of this is that how we move and how we physically present ourselves is reflective of who we are and how we respond on our emotional, mental, and spiritual levels. If we get a *good* massage from someone who knows what they are doing, at the very least we'll feel relaxed when it's over. In order for that to happen, tension has to be released. By definition, this means that emotions and thoughts have been eased or altered. We leave after the massage and realize our perspective has changed around certain issues.

All of these physical therapies I've mentioned (and the vast number of other such therapies I've not listed but that fall into this category) are geared to assisting and helping us to change by working with us through the physical level. That process can be as threatening as any other kind of therapy, and flower essences can be used to stabilize us exactly in the same manner I described for the counseling situation.

This concept may be a little difficult to believe, but the only thing I can say is that if you utilize a form of physical therapy in your life, either in a formal setting or at home on your own, try testing yourself before and after each session for about five sessions. I think you're going to be surprised to find all the things that are going on of which you weren't aware.

My personal experience is with Feldenkrais, a technique that is designed to teach us what limited or inefficient patterns of physical movement we've fallen into and alternatives to those patterns in order to give us physical options and agility as we move. About four years ago, I had occasion to have one of the top Israeli teachers work with me. To prepare, I tested myself for flower essences, and I was fine. I needed nothing. I went through an intense, yet very gentle, half-hour session with this man, who knew precisely what he was doing, and I left suspecting my entire body had been rearranged. I barely recognized the feelings of my own body. While waiting for a friend to finish her session with him, I retested the essences. I needed approximately eight essences. While he had worked, I unconsciously cooperated by shifting on all my other levels—and I had blown about eight circuits in the process. Taking the essences reconnected me and provided the support to integrate what he had accomplished on the physical level.

If you are a practitioner or teacher of any of these physical therapies, I urge you to incorporate the flower essences into your practice. After a session with an individual, as a general practice, give them the basic essence test and any essences that are needed, making sure they understand the definitions. The essences bring full circle and complete what you attempted to do in the session. And the client leaves in a state of balance and support and is more capable of integrating the changes that occurred during the session. Also, if you are working with someone and they want to make a change, and you see they need to make that change, yet it's not happening no matter what you try, stop the process right there and test for essences. Something deep may have surfaced and is sitting there creating a block. The essence helps identify the block/issue, which is the underlying cause for what you are working with, and temporarily gets the block out of the way so that you can continue with the physical change. In this case, identifying to both you and the client what is going on goes a long way in assisting that person to move through the emotional process that will remove the block permanently. Sometimes just hearing the definition does the trick for them. And taking the essence and having the electrical support while they move through physical change also serves as a stabilizer. In short, you're supporting them physically, electrically, mentally, and emotionally. This makes for a terrifically efficient session.

Just in case it's not as obvious as I think, let me also suggest that anyone who is a counselor or emotional therapist also incorporate the essences, testing the client prior to their leaving the office. This assures that the client is leaving in one piece, able to integrate what went on, and more able to deal with the world outside the therapeutic office.

To go further, it would be good to keep some empty dropper bottles and brandy on hand in case a client tests he needs certain essences for any period of time. Make a solution bottle, let them know how many days and how many times per day to take it, and be sure they know the definitions for their essences. (Also be sure they agree to your using the essences with them.) This way you as the therapist can help this person continue the beneficial effects of the session beyond the office.

TWO-WEEK ESSENCE PROCESS

This process is similar to the peeling process in that it deals with layers. But rather than peeling away many layers within a period of a half-hour as in the peeling process, the two-week flower essence process removes the layers more slowly — one layer or a combination of related layers per day.

It always delights and surprises me how smart we human beings really are. And this process is an excellent example of what I'm talking about. There are some issues that we file away on a long-term basis, and they are so integrated that they become a part of our everyday weave on every level. They are so much a part of us that they play a role in how we define ourselves, see ourselves. They are fully integrated patterns. And they impact us on every level.

For example, with regard to the physical, we will go through twenty or thirty years of our lives assuming that certain pain or a tendency toward structural weakness or a recurring health problem is there because "that's just the way we are." Then thirty years down the road, we start working with something like flower essences and changing our attitudes about our health and illnesses, and it dawns on us that we don't have to have certain health glitches if we don't want them. Usually we just get tired of the six colds a year or the weak left knee that gives out under a certain amount of stress or the chronic constipation or the twelve migraine headaches we know we can count on this year. Up to a certain point, we can integrate these things to such a degree that when they are triggered and pop to the foreground, we accept and endure them. At some point, however, they get irritating, tedious, and definitely in our way. When we scream, "I'm mad as hell and I won't take it any longer!" that's when we're ready to do something — and that's when the two-week flower essence process comes in.

Now, thirty years back when we started integrating this thing as part of our pattern, we didn't integrate the glitch. We integrated the reason for the glitch — the underlying cause. In this case it's usually a fear, a trauma, a circumstance that got internalized and, when triggered, gets externalized by way of the glitch. The causes tend to be serious issues. Here's where our brilliance comes in. Consciously we are not aware of the underlying issue. But when we finally decide to address the glitch it has created, our whole being, including our electrical system, steers us away from the fast-paced peeling process. Stripping the layers away and un-covering the core issue in this fashion is too much and too fast for us to handle. We need to address it more slowly. It's not just the seriousness of the core issue that is the consideration here. Don't forget that this is a long-term situation and the layers were not casually created. They have become as much a part of the integra-tion and weave of who we are as the core issue itself. So the two-week process *slowly* removes one layer at a time and allows us to adjust to that change before removing the next layer.

Figuring out if you need to do a two-week process takes a com-bination of common sense, reason, and intuition. If you have a migraine headache and your essence testing takes you only as far as the basic test—the peeling test doesn't come up, and when you tried telegraphing the migraine, you got that you were clear and that no essences were needed—that's when it will suddenly hit. You'll say something like, "Wait a minute. I have these things all the time. Something's going on here." That's your common sense, reason, and intuition functioning for you. Your intuition is saying, "Hold it Harriet/Harry!" Your reason is pulling in the fact that these headaches happen often. And your common sense is telling you something must be going on. So the next move is to ask:

Do I need to do a two-week essence test? (Test)

Bet you get a positive.

The two-week test is easy. All you do is the basic flower es-sence test one time each day (preferably morning) for the next two weeks. Be sure to test how many times that day you will need to take the day's essences. You do not need to test for number of days for each essence because you will be taking them for the one day only. You may get a repeat essence the following day, but this addresses the next layer. Whatever time of day you choose to test, make it consistent throughout the full two-week period. This will assure that you have a twenty-four hour period of time in which to release and integrate the change for each layer. The two-week process is complete when around the end of the two weeks you test clear, no essences needed. To double-check, ask:

Is this two-week process now complete? (Test)

If you get a negative, retest the essences to find what you missed and continue doing this daily until you get a positive. When you get a positive, you're done.

I fell onto this process a few years back when apparently it was time for me to get rid of a number of these old patterns, and I ended up doing one two-week process after another for a period of six months. As soon as I finished one, I was into the next one. So I learned something about the pattern these things take. First of all, I call it the two-week process because every one of them took exactly two weeks. And anyone I've tested to go on this process also took two weeks. I have no idea why there is consistent timing. But in telling you this, I would also like to pass along a warning not to assume this process will always take just two weeks. I've yet to discover an issue that took less or longer, but my gut feeling is that we should keep a sense of flexibility around this time issue.

Another pattern that was consistent had to do with the core issue. I always became aware of the core issue in the middle of the two-week period, not at the end. I kept a record of all the essences I was taking (something I highly recommend you do), and when I reviewed the two weeks, I saw that the first half of the process had to do with the peeling away and preparation I needed for the core issue. Then the core issue was identified, and the last half of the process focused on the healing and integration of the information I got from the core issue.

I also found that I was never able to get a hint of what the core issue was from the essences I needed prior to its identification. More often than not, they seemed totally unrelated, and I gave up trying to see a pattern that would tip me off as to what the core issue was. I suggest the same to you. It's a game we can easily fall into and, based on my experience, it seems to be a complete waste of time. Plus it can get in the way. We may think we've got an idea of what's coming, but we run the risk of distorting how we perceive the core issue once it does come up. The essences in the first half of the process seemed more directly related to the specific layers I was releasing and addressed the different patterns of protection I had cleverly devised.

I found I could not anticipate either what the core issue was or when it was going to pop up. At first I'd wait—a little like sitting around waiting for paint to dry. After all, this was important stuff, and the least I could do was give it the proper respect by waiting. Well, as if watching paint dry, I got real bored and eventually tossed this warped idea of respect out the window and got on with my day-to-day life. That's when I noticed the next thing that eventually proved to be another pattern. I would say that nine times out of ten, the identification of the core issue was triggered by some mundane, common, everyday occurrence. A person would tap me on the shoulder to say something and the tap would trigger the insight. Or someone would say something to me in a particular way. The wording would be the trigger. Or I'd absentmindedly tap a tree trunk as I walked by. And bingo, suddenly there it was in my mind.

Another point — and here's where I saw that human brilliance come into play again. If the core issue had to do with something I could personally handle well on my own, the trigger often came from a stranger or someone I barely knew, and the resulting insight would occur while I was in a larger, impersonal environment. When the insight was emotionally shocking or challenging, the trigger always came when I happened to be feeling safe and was with someone with whom I felt safe. I never experienced the insight of the core issue in an inappropriate or threatening environment. The same thing has happened with the others I've tested for the two-week process. I say this to you so that you can relax and know that if we don't stubbornly interfere, that natural protection device inside us will do its job, and we won't be left emotionally hanging out there in the wind.

About these core issue insights: I found that one second there was nothing, and the next second after the trigger, there was an instantaneous insight that usually popped up as a very clear, concise thought. It didn't come with a banner saying, "This is the core issue." But there was always a quality and clarity about it that immediately struck me as this being *it*. In short, what I'm trying to say is that as you move through your day, I don't think you have to worry about missing this insight. It just hits and there it is as obvious as an elephant doing the hula. It's going to be hard to overlook. In addition, the fact that you've even entered this process means you're all programmed and ready to get this insight. If you weren't ready, you wouldn't have addressed the glitch in the first place, nor would you have considered entering the process.

Often the insight came in the form of a flash — an insight that produced a clear emotion, a feeling, a taste, a visual picture,

186

either symbolic or actual. That is, another trigger would serve to move me mentally and emotionally into a specific direction. The fullness and clarity of the core issue would develop and flesh out as my thoughts moved in a free-flow manner in the direction that was triggered. Sometimes the core issue had to do with an old issue that I had already begun to deal with and put into balance, but it still needed a little more attention to add a final touch and complete the process. The fact that I initially tested the physical glitch was my way of saying that I no longer wanted the issue or its physical pattern as part of my life. So these particular types of insights were neither a surprise nor traumatic. Seeing how they paired with their specific glitches was certainly interesting.

But there were core issues that came as a complete surprise, and sometimes, not always, they were especially painful to look at. This was always when I was in a protected environment. I would look at the insight, follow it along in free-flow thought, sometimes feel pain around it that I had not recognized or felt before, perhaps cry, and in about a half-hour or forty-five minutes, I had moved through the insight. I have felt that part of the purpose of the essences taken for the week prior was in preparation for the time when I would need to look at and move through the insight. Although sometimes the process was difficult, I never had the feeling I was over my head or falling apart. And one last thought on this: I suspect that the time period needed to move through the insight depended on my willingness to move with it and not try to avoid it or buffer myself from the experience.

Another pattern: As soon as I was finished moving through the insight process, I tested the essences. Whereas the essences prior to the insight often left me in the dark, the essences taken right after the insight process was completed and for the rest of the two-week period had to do with recuperation, healing, rest, and integration. I knew I was through the comparatively short insight process by the fact that I would always have a terrific feeling of peace and comfort immediately following — no matter how difficult the last half-hour or so had been. But also I noticed that as I went through the rest of the days, different ideas would come to mind as to how this core issue wove into my life. I found these thoughts to be the completion part of the core issue process and very much a part of the healing, recuperation, and integration period.

Back to the physical glitch that got us into this in the first place. Most of the time I got so involved with the process and what I had learned from it that it would be weeks or months down the road before I realized, "Hey, that old pattern is really gone!" Just as those patterns had gotten all tied up in my life's weave in a subtle, unassuming, even quiet way, they left me in much the same manner. They just weren't there any longer. I'm talking about three to four months' time here. Sometimes I might have another "flare-up" of the glitch — this always occurred when the pattern was especially long-term and deeply ingrained — but it was never to the degree of intensity as before the two-week process. When the flare-ups occurred, all I'd have to do is test myself for essences, doing the basic test only. The flare-up would then subside immediately. It usually meant that my body and mind needed more time to establish new, more healthful ways to process whatever used to be processed through that old, more familiar pattern and glitch. But even the most difficult and deeply ingrained physical patterns were gone within a year's time.

There's one other issue I need to bring up, and that has to do with karmic issues we have brought from other lifetimes in order to clean up, clarify, and work them out in this lifetime. Often, those karmic issues will externalize physically and become part of the weave of our life and health. This makes sense. If we're going to go to the trouble of activating this kind of thing in order to further work on it, it would have to become somehow interwoven in the present life. Karmic patterns reveal themselves as core issues in the two-week essence process. What's happening here is that your irritation with the physical glitch and the decision to address it using the essences is you saying on that brilliant human level of yours, "It's time. I'm ready to look at this. Let's bring it up in a clear, conscious manner and see what we can do with it."

Without consciously realizing what we're dealing with, we go into the two-week process and get to a very strange insight. Now, in my experience, the thing that starts the insight is familiar and present-time to us. But as we move along in that free-flow state, this familiar situation begins to connect and associate with insights about events that are out of the present time. Suddenly you "see" yourself in the Middle Ages in Italy as a boy interacting with some domineering woman you recognize now to be your son. Don't attempt to censor these insights or thoughts, no matter how crazy they may seem. Allow yourself to move through the process with full attention on what you are either "seeing" or feeling. Mentally collect data. As you move through it, the core issue will reconnect back into your present life, and you'll be able to work through and integrate all the data into your present situation. In short, the core issue that is connected to the glitch you began testing had in itself a core issue that went back to another lifetime. And to fully complete the process, you needed to understand something about its origin.

A few words of warning about all of this: The two-week process is an extremely efficient and powerful tool to have at hand – obviously. I know that some people reading this will immediately say, "Oh great! Now I can clear out all my trash." But I warn you about making such a statement and arbitrarily acting on it. This all-out blitz approach denies that brilliant human aspect we each have inside us and ignores the important issue of timing that is so essential to the full success of the two-week process. We humans have free will. It sometimes manifests as stubbornness and stupidity. One of the things that gets us into trouble is our ability to override our personal timing. If we arbitrarily try to pull through a two-week essence process because of our idea that karmic "stuff" is to be cleared out right away, we will create more problems. When it comes time for the insight, that brilliant inner self will know that we are not ready to look at and assimilate this information, and we will experience the core issue in distortion. It's a protection. If we are hell-bent to pull through this process, all for the glory of eradicating our karma, of course, we run the real risk of misunderstanding the distortion or forcing some meaning into it when it really gave us no meaning, and getting sidetracked with some issue that is purely our own in-the-moment invention.

I think that the best way to avoid misusing the two-week process is to *always* test anytime we suspect we're to do it. Ask the question:

Am I to enter a two-week process? (Test)

If negative, back off and test the next time the idea pops into mind.

Or, go back to the physical glitch issue and let the body do the deciding for us. If we have discomfort but it really doesn't matter to us, it's not in our way, it's not that painful, it doesn't happen too often — if we can't say, "I'm mad as hell about this and I'm not going to take it any longer!" — don't test. That is, don't try to pull yourself through the two-week process. Instead, give yourself the basic test for the glitch for that one moment. You'll get the essences needed to stabilize you, get some relief, and maintain a holding pattern until that time when it's right to go into the two-week process. When the glitch becomes unacceptable, that's timing pulling our attention to the immediate matter of concern. In short, that's our inner timing saying, "Now."

Lastly, I have focused the two-week process on the issue of physical glitches. The same approach is used for emotional patterns and glitches. When a certain emotional pattern becomes unacceptable, when there's a stirring inside that suddenly draws our attention to this pattern and makes it seem like the biggest block in our life, that's the time to test to see if we are to enter a two-week process. Enter and move through the process in exactly the same way as I have described for dealing with physical issues. The principle is the same here; only the form of externalization is different.

Steps for the Two-Week Essence Process

1. Do the basic test and take the essences needed. Get the dosage information.

2. If you suspect a two-week test is needed, ask:
  Am I to do a two-week essence process? (Test)
If negative, back off and give yourself more time, but continue to do the basic test and take the essences as prescribed each time the physical or emotional issue arises.

3. If the result was positive, test yourself (using the basic essence test) one time daily for the next two weeks. Take the essences the number of times each day as prescribed. Keep a record of the essences taken each day. Ignore any multi-day dosage you got for the basic test essences in Step 1. The two-week daily testing supercedes this.

4. Allow the core insight to come through in everyday, mundane ways. When it comes, allow yourself to move in free-flowing thought, letting any thoughts or images come to mind. Don't suppress any emotions you might feel. Rather, make an effort to experience and identify them.

5. Do a basic essence test immediately after coming out of the core insight period. Then continue testing once a day until the end of the two-week period and you test clear. Ask:

Am I now clear in this two-week process? (Test)

If negative, retest to find the essences missed. Continue doing this daily until you test clear and also test positive to the above question. Then go celebrate.

CAUSES OF PAST PROBLEMS

You're getting the idea that you can use flower essences and the testing techniques I've been describing as a framework for getting specific insight on the cause-and-effect interplay going on in the body. Now you're curious. You used to have a problem, let's say stuttering, which was the cause of much concern and took great effort to get beyond. Although you no longer stutter, now you're curious as to what could possibly have caused that problem. It occurred prior to your present "age of essences," and as you progressed out of the problem, you obviously unconsciously made the adjustments necessary in order to strike the balance needed. Consciously, you have no idea of its cause. Or perhaps you have some suspicions. Now you want to know what was going on. Here's what you do.

Steps for Discovering Causes of Past Problems

1. Do the basic essence test and take any essences needed. Make sure you are clear. Get the dosage information.

2. Concentrate on the old problem. Rest your mind on the problem in general or on any one aspect of the problem that stands out to you.

This should take no more than a minute. If it's taking longer, you are either: 1) lost in the memory and need to return your focus to the fact that you wish to test this old problem and not relive it, or 2) unable to focus on the problem because it is still too painful and your mind is rejecting the memory out of a sense of protection. If it's the former, bring your mind back to what you want to do.

If it's the latter, consider not fighting yourself and put the idea of doing this test away for another, more appropriate time. If you willfully press on through the test, you run the risk of receiving insights and information that you aren't quite ready to integrate yet. You most likely won't know what to do with the information, and it'll feel like a strange, old bag hanging off your arm and getting in your way. For some information we need to feel safer and stronger than we presently are, so we need to educate ourselves to wait for the right time, the right place, and the right person with whom to share the experience of the insight. If you're wondering how to begin, developing the discipline to back off from this kind of testing when it's indicated that we should not continue on is one excellent way of gaining this necessary education.

3. When your focus is clearly on the problem, ask (aloud or to yourself):

Which essence or essences most clearly identify the underlying cause for this problem?

4. Test the essences and set aside or otherwise indicate which ones test positive. Read their definitions. Don't rely on your memory for the definitions. Usually, you will get just one or two essences in answer to this question. If you test positive for more, refocus on the problem, ask the question, and test again. Your focus may have been hazy. If you get the same results, consider your answer to be multilayered and complex, and proceed on.

5. Spend a moment thinking about the definitions, allowing your mind to move freely in the direction set off by those definitions.

6. Since this is a past problem, you do not need to take the essences for which you tested positive. In this process, they are being used for information and insight only.

That's it. You've got your information. The pieces should fall into place within ten to fifteen minutes. If after this time you're still unclear, put the essences away, keep the definitions in mind, and go about your day. As in the two-week process, something mundane will happen and all the pieces will fall into place.

Now the question is what to do with this information. Again, as with the two-week process, it can sometimes be surprising, even tough to look at. The cause behind a past difficult problem can't be unimportant. Yet I find that the answer often deals with something so close and familiar to us that its revelation often elicits a response of "I can't believe this." Don't toss the insight out as being not important enough. That's your logical self speaking, and you simply may not realize the depth of the impact this issue had on you. You may have to give yourself a little time before realizing the significance of the information.

I'll give you a personal example so that you can get an idea of how this testing works. A number of years ago, I had a uterine problem that I successfully worked through. One day after I began to use the flower essences, the question of what that problem was all about just popped to mind. I decided to test and followed the steps that I've outlined for you. The answer to my question was Zinnia Essence. Now, I don't make it a point to memorize the definitions of the flower essences, but I do remember the ones I use often—and Zinnia is an essence I use often. This time I felt the urge not to go on memory but rather to read the short definition.

Zinnia: Reconnects one to the child within. Restores playfulness, laughter, joy, and a sense of healthy priorities.

Here's where I discovered that, up to then, my mind had been playing an interesting trick. Whenever I had tested positive for Zinnia in the past, I kept reducing the definition down to "Damn it, I'm being too intense again and need to lighten up." This interpretation of the definition always worked for me. But for the test about the old, uterine problem, I felt the urge to read the short definition as written. The very first sentence, which I had always disregarded out of hand, suddenly struck me between the eyes. "Reconnects one to the child within." I sat with that feeling for a minute, and then I "saw" an infant in my uterus and realized *I* was that infant. The insight hit instantly that this was how I had protected myself from the child neglect and abuse that had begun when I was an infant. The place an infant would seek to go for protection is the womb. And since my mother could not physically accommodate me nor was she capable of emotionally accommodating my need for protection (she was one source of the problem), I literally enfolded myself in my own uterus. That is, I centered the stress I was under and the fear for my well-being as energy in my uterus. Apparently, all the pain and stress being held in the uterus could accurately be described and identified by the picture of the infant in the womb for protection. Hence, my insight. Also, in the insight, I *experienced* my adult body as having grown around this protected and enfolded infant in an even greater, buffer-like protection. There I was, an adult with an adult body that served to surround, buffer, and enfold the protected child within.

That protection was good and valid up to a certain point in life, and my body, my uterus in particular, maintained its health and balance. Then along came the diagnosed uterine problem. When I did the later essence test, I reviewed the timing of all of this and realized that by the time of the diagnosis, I had addressed the emotional issues regarding the abuse problem, gained in personal strength, grown to believe I could come out of myself and be safe, and I no longer had a need to keep the infant within. The protection had become unnecessary and inappropriate, and the uterine balance was lost. The combination of healing processes I chose in which to deal with the uterine problem enabled me to unconsciously release the child, to strike a new balance, and to restore the uterus back to health.

Coming back years later to find out what was going on was emotionally difficult. Having this information gave me a much deeper respect and love for myself. It also gave me an awesome insight into the human capacity to survive. I've come to understand that what I did as an infant is not an unusual reaction by infants who are in hostile environments. It saddens me deeply that this kind of thing happens to any infant, but it amazes me as well that an infant less than a month old can have such a creative instinctual survival response. So, difficult though this insight was, it has given me a deeper, broader understanding of and respect for myself and humanity in general.

I've told you all of this not because I have this deep desire to expose myself all over paper, but rather I want to give you an idea of the kind of information that can come up, the surprises it can offer, and the kind of enrichment you can receive from it. However, I do not feel that you should sit down and arbitrarily go through a checklist of every condition or problem you have ever had. I feel that, as in the two-week process, this kind of information needs to come to the surface in proper timing. After all, even though the insights may be unconscious, the problem has already been worked through, so it's not an immediate issue facing you. If you don't press and just make it a point to respond to the old issues as they naturally come to mind, you'll be better able to integrate and grow from the information you receive.

MORE ON CAULIFLOWER ESSENCE

I have already given the directions in the long definition for using the Cauliflower Essence for the newborn's benefit during birth. Since the Perelandra Garden Essences have been used by a bunch of folks, two issues have come up that need further addressing.

One. In watching the progress of newborns having had the benefit of the Cauliflower Essence during birth, it has become clear that the essence is stabilizing and balancing more than I originally thought possible. The Cauliflower Essence creates a bridge that connects the newborn with that which he has been prior to birth, even prior to conception, and with that which he is now—a spirit newly born into form. Before the use of Cauliflower Essence, this transition was so intense that we closed ourselves down during birth, thus creating a separation between what we were and have known and what we are now. A lot of time and effort is spent as we go through life attempting to open up to and reconnect these two existences of ourselves.

It is my understanding that the benefit of the Cauliflower Essence during birth is a new process and part of the many different changes we are now instituting into practice in order to assist a new generation coming into an environment of drastic change, challenge, and transition. It gives them the tools they will need to meet the challenges of their future. Consequently, although the Cauliflower birth process is beneficial and its time is right, it is still new. And the babies receiving this benefit now may need additional assistance to integrate into their newly born existence that to which they are remaining bridged. The Cauliflower Essence changes the dynamic of birth, and like anything that has changed or is new, there must be time for learning and additional help given during this time of learning. In short, even though this essence heralds in terrific and timely opportunity, it changes the game plan, and these new kids need a break while they rewrite the process a soul can expect to experience while going through birth.

The support for these newborns is easy. Complete the full Cauliflower birth process, giving the essence as prescribed through to the second day after birth. On the third day, give the baby a basic essence test. (*Always* be sure to test yourself first and take any needed essences so that you'll be clear before testing the baby.) If the baby tests clear, the integration is going well. Plan to keep tabs on how the integration is progressing by giving the baby a basic essence test once a week. Believe it or not, it is recommended that you do this for three months, the full amount of time needed for the completion of this integration process.

If the baby needed essences any time after the Cauliflower birth process was completed, test for the number of days and times per day the essences are to be given, administer them as prescribed, and do the follow-up basic testing. Newborns, as you might imagine, take a very light touch with the essences, and you might find one dose will do the trick. However, be prepared for the extremes of no essences or perhaps just one drop of one essence for the entire three months, or many drops of many essences given throughout — or anything in between. Each child will approach this integration issue differently.

A reminder about giving essences to newborns: Up to age three months, you can give a baby essences by putting one drop of each essence concentrate on the forehead. Then lightly rub the essence into the skin. You may also give the essences orally by putting one drop of each essence concentrate on the baby's lips, or if he/she reacts to the taste of brandy or you are uncomfortable about the brandy, dilute two drops of concentrate in 8 ounces of water and give the baby about ten drops of this solution.

Let's say you gave your baby the benefit of the Cauliflower birth process, but you were unable to keep tabs on the integration progress on a regular basis afterward. About three weeks after birth, a rash showed up. Guess who's having a little integration problem?! Whatever problem they are having is now manifesting physically as a rash. Easily taken care of. Just give the baby a basic essence test, administer any essences needed, and then follow up with a telegraph test for the rash. Administer those essences and find out how many days and times per day the rash essences are to be given. Each time you give the baby the rash essences, *you* will have to focus on the rash for the telegraphing, or you can "activate" the spot by touching it. After the prescribed period, do any necessary follow-up testing until the baby tests clear both with the basic test and the telegraph test.

Once the baby is clear, consider keeping a weekly tab for the remainder of the three-month period. You'll be able to catch problems before they have a chance to manifest physically.

One more thing: You gave the baby the Cauliflower birth process. You've diligently kept the weekly tabs for two months now and were just about to award yourself the "Boy!-Am-I-Ever-The-Best-On-Top-Of-It-Mom/Dad Award," and that little kid has the nerve to show some kind of weird symptom. Don't assume you failed. Assume your kid's clever and managed to sneak something by and, as will be with kids, is now suffering for his/her misguided efforts. Reach for the essences, give the basic test and any essences needed, then telegraph test the weird symptom and follow through as described above. Then give yourself the above-mentioned award.

Two. I said there were two things about Cauliflower Essence that needed to be addressed. Adults have been testing positive for this essence. And I mean men and women in their fifties and sixties, too. I'm getting letters: "I thought my ability to do the kinesiology testing was pretty good, but now I'm testing positive for Cauliflower, and, trust me, my name is Harvey and I'm not pregnant — and it's been sixty years since I was born."

Well, their testing *is* accurate. What is happening is that rather than having the bridge Cauliflower gives from birth, they have worked through their life to get to the point where it is appropriate for that bridge to be established now, and the conscious connection between "from whence they came" and "where they presently are" can be made. Hence the need for Cauliflower. Just as with the newborn, Cauliflower Essence will support and stabilize that connection process.

In this situation, don't do the Cauliflower birth process. Test for Cauliflower as a regular essence, taking it for the prescribed number of days as you would any essence.

ESSENCES AND THE DEATH PROCESS

One of the most helpful and constructive things we can do for someone as they move through their death cycle is to work with them with the flower essences. The focus now is not physical healing and health but rather physical, emotional, mental, and spiritual stability and balance.

I like to look at birth and death as two halves of one whole process, each half addressing different aspects within that larger, single process. So when we see a child being born, we see the second half of a process that actually began with a form of death—that is, the process of leaving one dimension for another. At death, we see the beginning of that process which, when beyond the death cycle, moves into birth—the process of arriving onto a new dimension.

With the Cauliflower birth process, we seek to support and stabilize the newborn's awareness of both the higher, expanded soul and the conscious child-soul as the two move through birth. During the death process, we do the same thing. Only now we are not dealing with a child-soul, and we are not actively supporting the arrival process, but rather we are supporting the departure process as well as the later arrival process. The goal is the same, however—to help the individual maintain conscious awareness during process.

When I first began using and studying the essences, it seemed most reasonable to me that they could be used to ease and stabilize people physically, emotionally, mentally, and spiritually as they faced death. It seemed that if ever there was a time to use flower essences, this was it. And if we wanted to respond with a sense of constructive purpose and direction to someone we love who was dying, flower essences were our tool.

Since the early days of study, however, I have learned more about the role of flower essences in the death process. I refer to that half of the process ahead of the person once he's died—the birth part, the arrival. The essences play a direct role in the stabilizing and support of the person once they have released from the body and are moving onto the new level. Physically, the soul maintains a direct link with its physical electrical system. The released soul energy, the soul reality, also contains within it a corresponding electrical system. So the essences given throughout the death process shift from the physical electrical system to the corresponding soul electrical system and serve to stabilize that corresponding electrical reality. This, in turn, assists and supports the soul on all its levels as it continues to move through the full process we call "death." In short, the person dying still has a need for physical support. Without it, he will feel as if the legs of a chair have been kicked out from under him. For just this reason alone, giving flower essences during the death process is more than beneficial. It is vital.

But there is more. When we leave this level of form (when we die), we do not suddenly disregard or forget what we just spent a lifetime learning—how we as souls function within a framework of form. To me, the logic of this is undeniable. Why bother going through all that time and effort experiencing life within the arena of form just to chuck the whole thing out the window the moment we die. When we die, our most immediate memory of ourselves as a functioning soul is within form. How we perceive ourselves and how we relate to all that exists around us continues to be through the window of form. To get a better idea of what I am saying, think of yourself as being suddenly displaced into a completely foreign country and culture. Everything is new. New language, new colors, new scenery, new currency, new food, completely new and different customs. To keep our bearings while we get used to all this new stuff, we will automatically go through the exercise of relating and comparing everything, including ourselves, to all the familiar things we just left. Sometimes we'll even recreate parts of the familiar so that the new environment won't feel so alien.

When we die, we do something similar. We maintain a memory of and a relationship to who we are as functioning souls within form. We may feel lighter, freer, stronger, more at peace, but all of this is perceived by us within the context of what we know best — our sense of form.

But it goes a step further. Our physical body "houses" our soul while we are experiencing form, and how well we relate soul to body during our life can be observed and measured by the state of our physical health. It's that inherent relationship between energy and form that I'm talking about. When the relationship is full, comfortable, and well-meshed, when the highest intent of the soul life is moving through its form, we see strength, health, and balance within the form. When the meshing is off, when something has happened to block that full movement of the highest intent of the soul through its form, we can see this misalignment as the form becomes unbalanced, weak, and dysfunctional.

After death, we go through a process of healing what remained unbalanced and dysfunctional within that lifetime. More often than not, we need only make a checklist of what went physically wrong that eventually led to death. This healing becomes our immediate concern once we have shifted and completed the full death process.

The most familiar avenue open to us for assessing how we are doing in this post-death healing and balancing period is our relationship to form. In death, we may leave the physical body, but its memory lingers on. And because the body has served as the barometer of the state and well-being of the soul expression, that memory of the body lingers on in the same state as the physical body we just left. Let me explain. If we died of heart trouble, the heart problem was the external sign of internal trouble. Once we pass over, we still carry the underlying internal problem which still affects how we perceive ourselves and how we feel ourselves to be physically. In other words, we can't possess the underlying mental, emotional, and spiritual imbalances on one hand, and then turn around and picture or perceive ourselves as being physically healthy on the other hand. The physical picture must jive with everything else. One automatically leads to the other. This direct relationship between energy and its resulting form is a basic universal law. The ability to imagine or perceive something in physical terms can only occur if there is correlating energy to support the physical imagery. Without it, you get a blank. If there is a distortion within energy, what becomes visible is the physical translation of that distortion. Cause and effect.

So, here we are, just having died from a heart problem. After a short "breathing" period—a bit like an orientation period—we realize that we must get on with the business of adjusting, balancing, and healing ourselves. So we enter a period of reflection and internal change. What better way to know how we are doing at any point along the way than to lean on the familiar and sense our "physical health." At some point we will turn around and say, "My heart is now healed." And we'll know that we have adjusted and altered ourselves to such a degree that we have eliminated all the underlying causes that had resulted in the heart problem. Only now are we capable of seeing, of sensing oneself as having a healthy heart. Energy and form are aligned.

How does all of this tie in with flower essences? you ask. First, I have been told that those who pass over after having had the benefits of flower essences during the death process "arrive" in far better condition than those who did not have essences. By "better condition" I mean in every way—emotionally, mentally, spiritually, as well as those aspects of us that still relate to the physical. Also, the brief "orientation" period goes much more smoothly for them. To quote: "They arrive miles ahead of the others."

Secondly, the person who has passed over continues to benefit from the flower essences that were given both in response to the illness and in response to the death process itself. The essences transfer, as it were, through the electrical system. Remember, the physical electrical system remains connected to and functioning with the soul reality and its corresponding electrical system through the entire process. As the person enters the reflection and change period, they are still being supported in those areas that are of immediate importance to them, which are directly related to the issues that dominated during the death process. I have been told that the healing process with those who have used flower essences during the death process is well under way by the time they enter the reflection and change period.

When to Use Essences for the Death Process

I am assuming a surrogate testing situation with this process, since, most likely, only the most determined of individuals will be able to keep testing themselves for flower essences while dying.

If the person is conscious, I feel it is essential to discuss the flower essences and offer your services, but let them make their own decision as to whether or not they wish to use the essences. Their sense of personal timing and appropriateness must remain paramount in this situation. Despite the benefits, flower essences just may not be what's right for them right now. However, I think you will be surprised at the positive response you get from the most unlikely of people when you approach them about the essences.

Case in point: My father was dying of cancer. He knew nothing about flower essences, knew nothing about my work and research with nature, he even knew nothing about my mind-set and philosophy of life. He did have this sneaky feeling that I was a little strange, however. The man could not have been more traditional in thought. Everything was strictly business within the context of the high-pressure New York business world. For the most part, our differences and our rocky history during my childhood made us more estranged than anything. I tell you all of this to illustrate the point that a positive response comes from the most unlikely of sources. This man could not have been more distant from the concept behind flower essences.

When I found out about his trouble and the probability that he would die from the cancer, I made the decision to phone and offer the flower essences to him. I would not argue their benefits, just tell him briefly what they were and what they did, and offer to test him if he wished. I fully expected a quick "no." Instead, he said "yes" and asked me to come to New York. I did this and tested him. I assumed he was half expecting me to come with a skull and crossbones, and a vial full of sacrificial goat's blood. He never winced once and he never asked what the hell I was doing with all that weird finger-pressing. He tested for the same two essences to be taken through the entire period of time he had left. I made a two-ounce bottle of solution and left it along with instructions, again assuming there was no way this man was going to take a few drops of the solution on a regular basis. I figured he was just happy I showed him some attention.

About four months later he called and asked for more of "that stuff in the bottle." Seems he ran out of the bottle I left him. I was stunned. For one thing, two ounces of essence solution taken a couple of drops at a time would last about eight months. The fact that the bottle was empty told me that he was taking the solution often. I said "sure thing," made another two-ounce bottle of solution, and sent it to New York. Here's the kicker. After he died (nine months after diagnosis and surgery), I was in his apartment and found the two bottles. The first one was indeed empty. The second one was completely full. For some reason known only to him, he chose not to take the essences through to the end. I have since learned that despite this decision, he still went through the death process and moved through that reflection, healing, and change period much more efficiently than if he had not had essences at all.

The moral to my story is for us to do our job of presenting the opportunity in a fair, clear, and honest manner, then to stand back and let them do their job of making a decision. I suspect strongly that at the time of death, those who wouldn't even consider such "hairbrained" things under normal conditions will very quickly and easily sense a positive opportunity and respond accordingly.

Now, if the person is unconscious or in a semi-coma, that's another matter. As I stated in *The Ethical Issue* in Chapter 7, this is something I feel must be approached carefully. The person's own sense of timing and appropriateness still must be regarded above all else. The easiest approach is to explain the essences to the person as if they were conscious. Assume they hear you. If they haven't died, they're still quite present. Then, after testing yourself and making sure you are clear, physically connect with them in some way. Resting their hand on your arm, wrist, or knee will do the job. Check your link as you would with any surrogate testing and then ask:

Do you wish to use the flower essences? (Test)

If it's a negative, I would back off and just lend my support in other ways as much as I could. If it's a positive, move forward with the testing.

Testing Flower Essences during the Death Process

I have found that the Perelandra Rose Essences, which deal with the various steps involved in process, are frequently tested for during the death process. If you see that you will be assisting someone (human or animal) during death, you might consider having this set of flower essences on hand along with any other essences you use.

1. Test yourself for essences and take whatever you need to clear for surrogate testing.

2. Do the basic essence test for the person and administer the essences. Be sure to get the number of days and times per day needed. Do telegraph testing for the major problems — for example, heart attack, liver cancer, the major issue that resulted in any surgery— the problems that are moving this person into the death cycle.

You do not have to telegraph test auxiliary problems that are a result of the major issue. Concentrate on the primary situation. If there was an accident in which the person was severely damaged in many different ways, concentrate the telegraph test and treat the accident itself as one, overall picture. However, if you have an accident victim with one or two major life-threatening problems and a bunch of auxiliary, more minor problems, concentrate the testing on the ones that are life-threatening.

3. Before leaving the telegraph testing, add one more test. For this one, you (as the surrogate tester) hold the question in focus. For most dying people it will be either too threatening or too emotional to focus on. Ask (silently):

> What essences are needed to stabilize him/her for the death process?

Then test the individual essences in the normal fashion, including the number of days and times per day the essences are to be taken. This test addresses and serves to stabilize the overall death-transition process itself, rather than all the individual components which are moving the person into the process.

Do the follow-up testing as indicated by first clearing the person with the basic test, then setting up for telegraph testing and asking the same question as above. *Important:* Even if you are not doing any other telegraph testing, either because the situation is too complicated or nothing other than the basic essence test is needed, do the telegraph test regarding the death process question.

If you have been testing the person all along in response to an illness, simply continue the follow-up testing through to the time of death. When it becomes evident to you that they have entered the death-preparation stage, add to your testing the telegraph test that deals with the overall death process. You'll either pick up on this switch intuitively, or you'll see a significant change in the essences needed, or the doctor will tell you.

About the definitions: I suggest common sense be used as to whether or not it will be helpful or harmful to the person to hear the definitions of the essences being given. Some people will be willing and even eager to have the essences during the pre-death period but will have a strong emotional reaction to hearing input that may relate obviously and directly to a situation that they prefer not to face head on—death. Yet there are others who will be relieved to have you interrelate with them in such a direct, straightforward way. So often the people surrounding them close down around the issue of death, leaving the person emotionally on their own. Having you share the essence definitions, the timing of the person's process, and the intimate knowledge of their fears and other emotions can be a terrific relief to them.

When faced with the issue of whether or not to read the definitions to the person, I'd let the person be the deciding factor. If this is unclear to you, try giving the definitions a couple of times and observe the person's reaction. Is it relief and curiosity, or is it dread, anger, or depression? The operating intent for you here is not to press beyond what the person wants. Insight as to underlying issues will be gotten later. Right now, the goal is to support and stabilize the person through transition.

4. IMMEDIATELY AFTER DEATH: If it is possible, do a basic essence test for the person within the first half-hour after death. Be sure you have cleared yourself with the essences before testing them.

Link with them, using your focus by visually concentrating on the body. Test to make sure you are connected. Then test the essences. If any essences test positive, this is what they now need as they move through this stage of the death process. Place one drop of concentrate on their forehead (first choice) or any other area of the body that is available to you. It is *not* necessary to lightly rub the essence in as you would for an infant. If the body is fully covered and you don't wish to disturb it, simply put one drop of the essence concentrate on the sheet or blanket covering the chest. This will put the essence into their immediate environment to be picked up by the electrical system. All of this post-death work is being shifted to the appropriate level and made directly accessible to the person through the electrical connection.

5. If it is at all possible, try to arrange that the body not be disturbed for three hours. This allows the person the full time period needed to completely detach from and move through the "birth" stage of the process. I know that if the person is in a hospital, you're going to have an uphill battle with this one. But you can get some of that time for the person by requesting that you (and/or the family) have time alone in the room before the body is taken away.

If the three-hour quiet period is not an issue and your presence is not needed for the sole purpose of buying the person the quiet time, you do not need to stay in the room. If you do, or if others wish to, it is best that everyone be as quiet and inwardly still as possible. This is not the time to express personal grief. You're still in the supportive role with the person as they move through the transition, and the focus needs to remain on them. After the three-hour period when the transition is complete, the focus can (and should) shift to personal pain, tears, and grief.

6. Before the body is moved, no matter how much quiet time they had, test the essences one more time using the basic test.

This last check is just to make sure the person is still stabilized as they move through the final transition stages. By this time, especially if you have been able to assist during the entire three-hour period, you will probably get an all-clear, no flower essences needed. If you don't, just administer one drop of whatever is needed on the person's forehead or on the covering over the chest area. This completes the essence process and the body can be moved.

If you have been able to move through the entire three-hour post-death quiet period, you will feel a distinct difference in the body from what you felt right after death. You'll have a very clear sense that the person is now no longer present around you and has truly gone on. Some people need less time to complete the full transition process. If the person was aware and prepared for death, this post-death transition can occur in a very short period of time—ten or fifteen minutes. You may feel a difference in the room and clearly sense that the person is no longer present. If that feeling is strong for you and you have no questions about it, do the last essence check at that point and then allow the body to be removed. (I am not taking into account here the time the people who love this person and who are present are going to need after the transition. I am only talking about the needs of the person who just died.) If you only suspect that the person has left or you just don't wish to act on gut feeling right then, allow for the full three-hour period, or for as much time as you can get for the person. In short, it is helpful for the person's transition if the body is left undisturbed for three hours. It does not interfere with or disturb the person if the body is left undisturbed for a period of time *after* the transition is complete.

HINTS: I suggest strongly that throughout the death preparation, death, and death transition process you check yourself for flower essences frequently to make sure that while you're in this role of the supporter, you are stable and supported. Also, after everything is complete, test yourself again just to make sure you are doing okay with this rather awesome experience.

If there are family and friends surrounding the person during this period of time, it would be helpful to them, to the person dying, and to you if they were checked for essences throughout. Everyone will be able to move through the process with a sense of support and inner strength rather than feeling like they have overloaded or short-circuited and are bouncing off the walls.

A word of encouragement to you who would like to assist someone through the full death process but for one reason or another were either stopped halfway through the process by someone or kept out of the picture altogether. It's okay. Think about the obvious. Lots of people have been dying successfully for a long time without the aid of flower essences. It is true that the essences allow us to move through the process more efficiently and with greater awareness and ease. What with the introduction of the Cauliflower birth process and the essence support for the death process, it looks as if it is the right time to broaden our experience during these transitions. But not having the essences isn't going to stop people from doing what they need to do in order to be born and to die. So a lost opportunity with someone we love is only just that — a lost opportunity. In this instance, your intent and desire to help, support, and assist with the essences will in itself be supportive and strengthening.

FLOWER ESSENCES AND ANIMALS

Using flower essences with animals is very easy, not to mention beneficial for the animal. For one thing, animals don't go through the process of complicating their illnesses and problems with an overlay of emotions within emotions like we humans do. And their physical body is set up to function in a similar manner to ours. Flower essences operate in their body in exactly the same way as in our body—only with animals it's less complicated. When I work with animals, I feel as if the nervous system and the electrical system are both right on the surface just waiting for the flower essences.

We use the essences with our animals any time they are sick, injured, in need of surgery, when there's an unusual behavior change, and in preparation for death. The only testing procedures we use are the basic essence test and telegraphing. The essences help our animals move through illness or injury with speed and efficiency, even when used in combination with medicines or procedures prescribed by our vet. It's that electrical/nervous system support combined with and moving in tandem with the physical/medical support that does the trick.

Using Kinesiology

Kinesiology as a testing tool works with an animal's system exactly as it works with ours. A negative creates an overload or break in the circuitry. And a negative response to a yes/no question creates a break in our testing fingers. With a positive, their circuitry and our fingers hold.

To set up a test with an animal, you will do surrogate testing and set up as you would with a child. *Important: Be sure you test and clear yourself for essences before doing any testing work with animals.* You hold the testing focus, especially for any telegraph testing. Concentrate on linking with the animal and test to make sure you are linked before doing any testing. The animal does not need to be awake for this and, in fact, testing while they are a-sleep eliminates their squirming and getting distracted with every-thing going on around them.

I approach kinesiology with animals with the assumption that, as with a child or comatose person, words may be said and not be consciously understood, but the intent behind the words is com-pletely understood. At these times verbal words are but mere vehicles for transporting that intent to a human or animal. I also approach the testing with the assumption that all of nature is in-telligent and fully capable of giving accurate responses to *intel-ligible* questions. All we need is the means for translating those responses. That's where kinesiology comes in. So throughout the entire testing process with an animal, I will use the same precise, simple, yes/no-type questioning I use with humans. As with humans, the accurate, intelligent response isn't coming by route of the mind and mouth, it is coming electrically. My intent during the testing is to be in communication with the animal as a wholis-tic system capable of discerning that which is balancing and life-enhancing for it from that which is not.

Testing during Illnesses

If the animal is generally low or basically not feeling well (and because it's not serious enough to warrant a visit to the vet, we don't know precisely what's going on) just link with the animal and do the surrogate basic essence test. Find out what essences are needed, for how long, and how many times a day they are to be given. Animals, like children, respond well to the lightest of touches with the essences. It's rare that we have to administer the essences more than one time each day of the dosage period. Do any follow-up testing that is indicated in order to assist and support the animal through the entire recovery period.

For illnesses that have specific, "nameable" problem areas such as a lung problem, enlarged heart, or arthritis, do a telegraph test for those areas just as you would surrogate test a human. Do the basic test first and administer the essences; then concentrate on the problem areas one at a time, giving the essences needed for each area as you go along. Don't forget to get the number of days and the times per day for the essences needed for each area. And do any necessary follow-up testing. When administering essences for specific areas or problems, be sure to link with the animal and hold the focus for each area as the essences are given. This will telegraph the essences into the correct area.

Testing for Fleas

This isn't an illness, except for the headache given to owners, but it is something for which you might try using essences. We have found that the amount of fleas on an animal and the general health and balance of that animal are related. The stronger and more balanced the animal is, the fewer the fleas. If your animal has fleas, try establishing a stronger balance by using essences.

First do the basic test to clear the animal, then telegraph test by asking:

What are the imbalances in this animal that are responsible for attracting the fleas?

Test the essences, then test for days and times per day. Don't be surprised if you have to administer the essence(s) throughout the entire flea season. (Make one great big, well-preserved solution bottle for the whole season.)

We have had limited success with this, and I think it is because we live in an area with such a high flea population that there is no animal alive with the balance to completely ward them off. I feel, however, that essences alone might be just the trick for animals who are not living primarily outdoors and in a woods. And even if the essences don't do a complete job, they are helpful and can be used in conjunction with other methods.

About other methods: Flea collars, spray, baths, tablets . . . We use kinesiology to find out which methods and which ingredients do not weaken or harm and which are most compatible for each animal. We don't make a blanket decision for all our animals based on the testing of just one. The balance we seek is to control the flea (and tick) problem, which can be a serious health problem if left alone, while at the same time maintaining the over-all healthy balance of the animal. This can be done by placing each item you wish to try on or near the animal and asking:

Is this (item, collar, spray, tablet) compatible with the animal's health and balance? (Test)

You can ask any more questions you might have as long as they are worded in a simple yes/no format. If you end up with more than one that is compatible, use whichever you prefer.

Testing When There Is a Change in Behavior Pattern

Noticing a change in an animal's behavior pattern is about as clear an early-warning signal as we can hope for. It can indicate the early stages of illness. If acted on quickly enough, doing the basic essence test (only the basic test will be needed) and giving the animal those essences can prevent the situation from deteriorating into illness.

A change in behavior can also indicate that an animal is having difficulty with some emotions that are flying around the house. Animals are affected by our emotional energy, especially when it is unprocessed, unresolved emotional energy. They are very like children in this regard, in that both will absorb the emotional energy around them and either begin acting out in response to these emotions or hold them in and become sick. If this is hard to believe, just watch your pet for a couple of days after a difficult emotional exchange with someone else in the house, especially an exchange that remains unresolved and has led to silence between the two of you. Watch what your animal does. Nine times out of ten, you'll see a distinct behavior change. An affectionate animal will suddenly become distant. Or a normally aloof animal will suddenly want to be close. A lot of times, there will be hyperactivity.

Link with the animal and test it for flower essences. For this, you will also only need to do the basic essence test. When you see the essences that are needed, you'll recognize that they have a direct relationship with the emotional issue between you and the other person, and have nothing to do with the animal. In this situation, give the animal the needed essences for the prescribed period of time — and, if possible, take the hint and work to resolve the emotional issue. If this can't be done right away, keep an eye on the animal's behavior and test again if you notice any more changes.

I mentioned this in *Behaving* . . ., but I feel it should be repeated here. This has to do with people who work in a service designed to bring to the surface and release other's emotions. That would include counselors, therapists, and clergy, as well as physical therapists and massage therapists. If you have an animal around the office, it would be a good idea to test it for essences frequently — at least once a week. Chances are excellent that the animal is a virtual sponge for the emotional energy that is released and left by each client. After an animal takes on this emotional energy day after day after day, its health and well-being will be adversely affected. Again, I realize this may be difficult to swallow, but if you have an animal in an environment such as this, test it a few times as an experiment and just look at the results. They will verify what I am saying.

For Injury

Do exactly as you would do for a human with an injury. Do the basic test. Administer the essences. Then telegraph test each injury, making sure you get the dosage information. Do the follow-up testing until the animal tests clear, and no further essences are needed.

For Overnight Stays at the Vet and Surgery

None of our animals enjoys going to the vet, even though we have terrific, kind, concerned vets. Our animals don't seem to be overly impressed with this and get very unhappy about the whole ordeal. They especially aren't too pleased with the idea of having to spend the night, a very rare occurrence. If we know or even suspect that the vet might want the animal overnight for tests or surgery, I prepare them by checking for essences. This may seem to be an indulgence to the animal, but if they are spending the night, something serious is going on, and I don't want their fear of being in an unfamiliar environment to complicate the situation.

Once the animal is at the vet, they're out of my hands. So I do an essence test just prior to leaving to prepare for a possible overnight and/or surgery. I do the basic essence test, giving any essences needed. Then I telegraph test two questions:

Are any essences needed if _____ has to spend the night at the vet? (Test)

If yes, I test and administer those essences, then ask:

Are any essences needed in preparation for surgery? (Test)

If positive, I test and give these essences, as well. And off we go to see the vet.

After I get them back home again, I put them on essences if they are sick or injured and continue the testing through the entire recovery period. For surgery, I use the essences to help them heal and recover, and I test through the entire period.

All of this testing may seem terribly tedious, but you'll find that animals use essences in a less complex way than we use them. You won't be testing animals every day; instead, it will be more like every week or two. And the number of essences needed will tend to be less. It's just important to understand that we need to support and assist an animal throughout the entire healing and recovery period just as we would a human — only with animals, it's not so much work!

Administering Flower Essences to Animals

There are several ways to administer the essences to animals. If the daily dosage coincides with mealtime, one drop of concentrate for each essence can be put on the food. If the essences are to be given more than once daily, you can put 3 drops of each essence into a bowl with 6 ounces of water. Another easy method is to make a solution bottle that has a plastic dropper with it and administer the essences directly into the mouth. Wash the dropper before putting it back into the solution bottle. You can either put two drops of each essence concentrate into a one-ounce solution bottle or, to be more precise and economy-minded, test the essences separately as you would normally to get the exact amount needed per ounce.

Flower Essences and Animal Death

This is the situation I usually get asked about when it comes to animals. By definition, a pet or companion animal is a friend, a member of the family. Letting go of that friend can be as difficult as letting go of a person we love. By taking advantage of the quality veterinary and health care we have available, it isn't unusual to have an animal as part of our lives for fifteen, maybe twenty years. That's longer than a lot of marriages these days.

When facing pet death, we have several issues coming in on us simultaneously. 1) This is our friend. Sometimes, this is our longest-lived and closest friend. 2) Our friend can't communicate in the "normal" way, so we can't sit down and discuss their wishes as to medical process and procedure. And by the fact that this animal is a pet, he looks to us for everything needed for survival. He is in some ways as dependent as a baby. 3) Veterinary medicine gives us about as much option medically as our own medical structure – and as expensively. Where we used to keep Fido warm and quiet until death after being hit by a car, veterinary medicine can now restore him to health. 4) Veterinary medicine offers euthanasia as a legal and viable option. This throws us right into the middle of the "death with dignity" controversy.

By the time people ask for my advice, they are pretty much frazzled by the impact and emotional cost of dealing with all four of the above issues, usually all at the same time. They have a clear idea that this pet, although an animal, is of value and not something to just be killed and tossed out when care becomes too troublesome.

Within the past three years at Perelandra, we've had a number of our animal friends pass on. We've lived here long enough for the puppies, kittens, and other baby animals we got fifteen years ago to live a full life, enter their "senior citizen" days, and pass on. It's never easy emotionally. That's a given, and we who have animals in our lives might as well reconcile ourselves to this fact. When the animal dies, it's going to hurt. Period. There will be a period of grief and adjustment, no matter how stiff our upper lip is. I find often that people make their pets go through a terrible, drawn-out, and difficult time by relying on their vet to keep the animal alive solely because they (the owner) do not want to face the emotional pain of loss. This is a terrible burden to give to the animal.

The grief issue has become so recognized that some vets have on staff a grief therapist who does nothing but assist the owner/friend once the animal has died. After the death of our sixteen-year-old cat named Fred, our vet told us how difficult it is for him these days to see all the puppies and kittens he treated fourteen years ago when he began practicing now come to an age where many have lived out their lives and must be "put to sleep." He said that in veterinary school, they don't deal with the issue of the pain experienced by a vet when an animal they've treated for so long dies or needs to be put down. And they also don't talk about how to deal with the pain and grief of the owner during such times. Consequently, vets may be clear that an animal can no longer sustain a reasonable life and has reached the end of the line, but they may have little knowledge of what to do to help a person face this loss of a friend. Reactions can be quite extreme. Like the time our vet had to tell an ex-marine that his dog needed to be put down as soon as possible — and the rather large, well-developed ex-marine fell apart right on the spot.

Why am I telling you all of this? Well, I feel this grief business is made that much worse when we feel conflict over the depths of what we are feeling and the fact that we are feeling it for an animal. Some people know beyond question that this is a friend. Others get into a push-pull dilemma and resist the emotions, thinking that "regular" people just don't have these feelings about an animal. Well, it's something felt by everyone, including the animal's vet.

I get involved in this because often I find that the primary thing keeping people from thinking clearly about how to assist an animal through death is their reluctance to accept the sorrow of separation and the inevitable grief. It clouds our ability to make clear decisions based on what is best for the animal. One thing to remember about animals is that they are not at all sentimental about death. From my experience with assisting them during the death process, I feel that they see death as a natural part of life and, if we allow them, they will move through it with extraordinary grace.

What I encourage people to do and what I do myself is put effort into separating my feelings of personal pain around losing this friend from what needs to be done for the sake of supporting that friend throughout the pre-death and death process. I try my best to make decisions based on what is good for the animal. If it means I will take an emotional hit, so be it. My focus is on the animal and what I am to do, as his friend, to give him the support and quality of life and death *he* wants and needs. In short, I try my best to keep my focus on the best course of action for the animal.

If the animal has obviously entered the death process and is moving through it in comfort, I will link with the animal and ask if medical assistance is needed and/or wanted. If I get a negative (which has usually been the case), I will keep the animal physically comfortable and in a quiet, private area. I've seen that animals prefer privacy during this time. In fact, when I suspect that death for an older animal can't be too far off, I watch them for signs of their seeking privacy as an indication that they are now entering the death process.

I do have personal issues about the quality of my response during the death process and I make these issues very clear to the animal. I tell any animal I am assisting that if it is unable to eat or drink in the normal fashion but could eat or drink if I assisted, I will assist. I will not deliberately let it starve to death nor will I let it become dehydrated, unless the animal is in such bad shape that ingesting food or water would be completely inappropriate. I personally have difficulty not responding to an animal in need of food or water. I make it a point to be clear about this because if the animal was "planning" to quietly starve to death, I'm not going to let that happen. It's beyond my personal code of ethics and I feel I have a right to that code, as long as it's reasonable. The animal will have to quietly die in another fashion and I will assist them, if necessary. In my experience, I have never felt that my refusal to be a party to starvation or dehydration has interfered with the animal's timing in any way. To the contrary, I've felt that by being clear about this, the animal was able to make any appropriate adjustments needed for its process.

I think the really difficult experience with animal death is when the issue of euthanasia enters. This puts the decision for death right into our laps, and that's real uncomfortable. Clarence and I base our decision on three considerations: 1) the information and advice of our vet, 2) the quality of the animal's life if we work to sustain it, and 3) the "desires" of the animal itself.

First of all, we have a couple of vets we have grown to trust through the years, and we have encouraged them to give us as much information about the condition of our animals as we can understand. In many ways, they have given us a terrific education, which has included letting us look at samples under the microscope and examine x-rays taken after injury. So, when we come to that moment of decision about putting down an animal, they know we want to hear everything about the animal's condition and have the benefit of their (the vet's) opinion.

Secondly, I feel strongly that animals have a life quality and a right to live life with that quality. Just breathing, laying in a corner and watching traffic go by, to me is not an animal's life quality. If they were in the wild, weakness, old age, injury, and illness would be dealt with through quick death or being killed. But we can protect and sustain them. Sometimes that means they have a chance to heal, recover, and continue on with a full or partially disabled life. At other times it means we can put them into a death-like existence. Sometimes it's a fine line between the two.

I watch for personality changes that indicate to us that sustaining them has now become an irritation to them. For example, we had a pet skunk (named Louie) who, in his later years, developed a deteriorating spinal column. He slowly lost mobility in his hind legs and, eventually, his entire hind end. He wasn't in pain, and after consulting the vet, we decided to let Louie continue on as long as his life gave him pleasure. In the wild, his lack of mobility would have made him easy prey and he would not have been faced with decisions of this sort. But because we were involved, his life took on a greater complexity. For awhile, he continued to enjoy walks in the woods each day. Then he enjoyed drags in the woods—he didn't seem to care that his hind legs weren't working. He spent more time in the house with us, and we realized it was for both company and the fact that he could easily pull himself around the slick floors. The woods' floor was becoming as issue with him. Then his desires and personality changed. He no longer wanted to come out of his den. He only came out to eat and then he'd go right back in. He was irritated anytime we opened the den to see how he was. He wasn't living, he was existing. As long as we gave him food and water, he could continue existing. It was then we made the decision it was time to put him down.

The first thing I did was to tell him (literally) that this was our decision. I did this to set up for a kinesiology test. I then asked him:

Do you wish to pass on now? (Test)

I got a strong yes—Louie was always a blunt, straightforward fellow. Then I told him exactly what we planned to do and that it would include a trip to the vet. I told him about the shot he would receive and what it would do to him. I then asked:

Do you agree with this course of action? (Test)

Again another yes. I asked:

How many days do you need to prepare to die?

I tested the number of days sequentially, beginning with:

1 day? (Test)

2 days? (Test)

3 days? (Test)

4 days? (Test)

As soon as possible? (Test)

I got a strong yes on the last test. Clarence made an appointment with the vet for the following day. And I told Louie when he would be going to the vet. Then I tested him for essences to see if he needed anything as he prepared. As it turned out, Louie needed Royal Highness (Perelandra Rose Essence), the essence for "final stabilization. The mop-up essence which helps to insulate, protect, and stabilize the individual and to stabilize the shift during its final stages while vulnerable." Louie was to receive Royal Highness one time that day and one time the following morning.

Just before going to the vet, I tested him again. He was fine. I reminded him what was going to happen and told him we would be bringing his body back to Perelandra for burial. I also told him we would be giving him the full three-hour transition period for his separation process prior to burial. This way he would know he need not be concerned with anything but transition and that we would still be there in a supportive role. And I asked him one more time:

Are you ready for death? (Test)

I got a strong yes.

I go through all of this clarity and explaining business because it keeps the entire process clear and clean for both us and the animal. My verification of this is what occurs at the vet. This is the toughest part of the process for us. We always handle and hold our animals when the vet administers the shot. As I mentioned before, going to the vet is never a happy time for our animals. They all establish their personal patterns of resistant behavior over the years. In every case, when we have had to put them down, they changed that pattern dramatically. Each animal was quiet, calm, and sometimes even helpful. Our dog, Jesse, lifted her paw for the injection. To us this consistent change in behavior has been a clear indication that indeed these animals were prepared and ready to go.

In case you are curious, let me tell you about our experience at the vet at the moment of death. Our vets inject a massive over-dose of phenobarbital into a vein, usually in the foreleg. Some-times they have to shave a small patch of hair from the foreleg in order to more easily locate and inject the vein. This is especially true when the animal's blood pressure is low. Within seconds, I can feel the animal's body begin to relax. I'll use my hands to gently guide them down to the towel we placed under them before we began. Although I am usually speaking to the animal in a low voice, encouraging him to relax, and assuring that every-thing is fine, this has been a very quiet and gentle moment. We wait a couple of minutes, then the vet will check for heart activity, verifying death. We spend perhaps another twenty minutes or so in the room, all of us quietly talking, usually reminiscing about our friend, while getting our hearts back out of our mouths. Some-times the animal will twitch or move during this time, but this is just the body and its nervous system naturally letting go. It can be a bit weird to see if you're not prepared for the possibility. Then we wrap the animal in the towel and take him back to Perelandra for burial.

Our experience with this, although tough emotionally, has always been special. I think it is good for our friend to die in loving and caring hands, and I think it is good for us to experience the peace and tranquility of the moment.

I know not all vets are as compassionate as ours toward both the animal and the owner, and some prefer to put an animal down without the owner present simply because it's easier on everyone. I think this is especially true if we owners are not going to be able to maintain a calm composure during the process. Hysterics won't help anyone. But if you are inclined to experience this time with your animal, you can request to be present and the vet will agree. Also, if you have property and wish to bury the body there, you can make arrangements with the vet to receive the body back even if you are not present for the injection.

Now, we still have the burial part of the process to go through. As I said, we bring our animals back to Perelandra. We leave them wrapped and in a quiet spot for three hours. As soon as we get the body back home, I clear myself with the essences, then I'll link with the animal—just as was described when linking with a human who has just died—and test again for essences. Several of the animals needed Royal Highness again. Louie didn't need anything. For those needing essences, I simply put a drop of concentrate on the wrapped body around the chest area. Then we leave them undisturbed for three hours. We don't make an issue of whether or not the other animals see or sniff the body. We leave that up to them and allow them to move through this period and the burial however they wish. (By the way, wild animals need only an hour for their post-death transition process.) As a matter of course, I test the animal one more time just prior to being moved for burial. Only once were essences needed.

By the time of burial, we have always been able to sense, to literally feel, that the soul of the animal has fully separated from the body and moved on. The body has the distinct feeling of being an empty vessel. In many ways, I feel like this entire process we've gone through has led up to the moment of placing the body into the ground and feeling beyond a shadow of a doubt that our friend has truly moved on and that the body is no longer needed. To me, just to have that stable, clear feeling at the burial is worth all the steps, testing, explanations, and rechecking.

At this point, I concentrate on my own grief process, my own feelings of separation. Within a few days, I can feel I've come through a painful passage and have come out the other end.

For essences, I test myself once a day while moving through the pain. I also will test the other animals the day following the burial to make sure they are adjusting in balance. Our animals always show signs of missing the one who has died, and I'll watch this to make sure they move through this period for themselves. If they appear to be "stuck," I'll test for essences.

Steps for Using Flower Essences
during the Animal Death Process

FOR A NATURAL DEATH:

1. As the animal moves through the pre-death period, do the basic testing (after testing and clearing yourself first) and administer the needed essences. Find out the number of days needed and times per day.

2. Telegraph test the question:
   What essences are needed by this animal to prepare for
   death? (Test the essences.)
Find out the number of days needed and times per day.

3. Do the follow-up testing for both the basic and the telegraph
test as indicated when each dosage period ends.

4. As soon as possible after death, test and clear yourself, then
link with the animal and verify that link by testing. Do the basic
essence test only. Administer one drop of each essence needed on
the chest area or the towel covering the chest area.

5. Wrap the body if that hasn't already been done. Place in a
quiet spot for three hours (pet), or one hour (wild animal).

6. Just before burial, test again (make sure you are clear first)
and put one drop of any needed essences on the wrapped body.

7. Bury the body. A suggestion: Cover the body with a thin
layer of lime (around 1/2") before putting the dirt on. The lime
will help with the decomposition of the body and will eliminate
decomposition odor.

FOR QUICK DEATH CAUSED BY INJURY:
1. Test yourself, the basic test only, and take any essences
needed.

2. Link with the animal, do a basic test, and administer the essences. Putting one drop on the lips will do fine if the animal
won't drink or take a dropper.

3. Telegraph test the question:

What essences are needed to stabilize this animal for death? (Test the essences.)

Administer those essences. If the animal remains alive for more than two hours, check again then, and every two hours up to death on whether or not the animal needs another drop of the essences needed to stabilize him for death. Do this by linking with the animal and asking:

Are the stabilizing essences needed again? (Test)

If positive, administer them. If negative, plan to check again in two hours.

4. When the animal has died, go through the death and post-death process as outlined in *Natural Death*, starting with Step 4.

NOTE: If you find your animal already dead and you suspect that death occurred within the past three hours, you can do one basic test for the animal and the essences will still be beneficial. After three hours, the animal has already separated from the body, and you won't be able to link yourself or the essences properly.

FOR DEATH INCLUDING EUTHANASIA:

1. Get full information on the situation from your vet, including what lies ahead if the animal continues to be kept alive. Consider your own feelings in the matter based on this information.

2. Clear yourself for testing. Link with the animal and ask:

Do you wish to die now? (Test)

We have never gotten a 'no' to this. If you do, ask:

Do you wish us to keep you living longer? (Test)

If you get a 'yes,' then you'll have to consider this when making your decision. This may come up if the animal is young but injured or ill, and the vet isn't sure about the outcome. The animal wants to fight for survival. However, by the time the vet has clearly suggested that the animal be put to death, we have always found that the animal already is fully aware of the situation and waiting to go. You won't be getting into an argumentative situation here with the animal. What you are doing at this point is maintaining clarity and verifying that clarity. You are not setting up a debate.

3. Make a final decision based on the vet's input, your feelings, and the animal's input. Whatever the decision, inform the animal what it is. The key for the animal's peace of mind and peace of process is clarity. Include the plans concerning the vet, the shot and what the animal can expect to experience with the shot (your vet can give you full details about this), and burial plans. (My sense is that they are able to adjust the transition process to however the body is treated after death. If you plan for the vet to keep the body for disposal, that is a very different situation for the animal from your bringing the body home for the three-hour transition period and burial. The animal doesn't care to make a judgment on this decision. But if clear on what is to occur, it will adjust its post-death process accordingly.)

Then ask:

Do you agree with the course of action I've chosen? (Test)

Again, based on everything I know, you're not going to get into an argumentative situation here either. However, if you do get a 'no,' ask:

Do you wish to die naturally? (Test)

If you get a positive, that's the animal's wish. If there is suffering involved, you can choose to not have the animal experience this, even though it seems to be acceptable to the animal. In this case, tell him that you won't be able to handle his suffering and wish for him to be given the injection. Then ask:

Is this acceptable? (Test)

You'll get a yes now. This animal is your friend.

4. Ask:

How many days do you need in order to prepare to die?

No additional time is needed?

1 day?

2 days?

3 days?

And so on with the sequential count until you get the amount of time needed. Because of their innate sense of the natural cycle, including death, and their lack of sentimentality around death, you'll most likely test from them that they are ready to go at any time. Once you know the schedule for the vet visit, be sure to tell the animal. (Remember, you are asking how many days *he* needs to prepare, not how long *you* need. Testing for essences throughout will keep you stabilized.)

5. Telegraph test the question:

What essences are needed to stabilize this animal for death?

(Test the essences.)

Administer these essences as prescribed up to when you leave for the vet's office.

6. Just before leaving for the vet, link with the animal and telegraph test the question:

Are you ready for the death transition? (Test)

A positive means all is ready. A negative means you need to do another essence test—just the basic test at this point will do fine.

Give the essences and ask if the animal is now ready. You'll get a yes now.

It would be a good idea if you test yourself before leaving for the vet, and test anyone else who's going along, as well. At least a basic test. But it would be better if you telegraphed the question, "Am I ready for this experience?" This extra step will help you while at the vet's.

7. Move through the post-death part of the process just as outlined in *Natural Death,* starting with Step 4.

FLOWER ESSENCES AND PLANTS

I'm going to fudge on this. Flower essences are useful for helping to establish plant balance, but there is also an entire approach to establishing overall plant balance which I have described and outlined in detail in the *Perelandra Garden Workbook.* If you are interested in working with plants and incorporating the flower essences, I suggest you get the *Workbook.* Once you have considered all of the various elements that go into creating plant balance, you'll easily be able to include flower essences. Plants, like all other life forms, need more than flower essences for full health and balance — like good soil, proper light, water . . . To include flower essences, be they house, garden, or landscaping plants, here's what to do. (These instructions will make more sense to those who have read the *Workbook.*)

1. Connect with the deva of the plant you wish to test.

2. Ask:
Does this plant need any flower essences? (Test)

If you are gardening and working with a row of the same variety of plants, you can ask the deva if that variety needs flower essences. If so, you'll be applying the essences to each plant in the entire row.

3. If you test positive to the above question, test the bottles of flower essences exactly as you would normally. Only this time you are linked with the plant via its deva. Also test for number of days. You need not test for times per day, since essences are applied to plants just one time daily, before 10 a.m. Normally, you will have to apply them for no more than one day. Perhaps one out of ten times you test, you'll need to apply the essences for more than one day.

4. Ask if the essences are to be applied by spraying the leaves or directly into the soil. Make a solution that will give you enough for whichever method you are to use. Once you choose the container for the solution, ask how many drops of concentrate are to be used for a container that size. (Don't be surprised if to two gallons of water you need only two drops of each essence concentrate. Plants don't need to be belted with this stuff.)

5. Apply the essences according to the tested-for means prior to 10 a.m.

To be honest with you, if you go through the various processes described in the *Workbook* and establish a balanced, overall plant environment, you will rarely need to use flower essences. I used them in the beginning of my gardening adventure some eight to ten years ago, but as I incorporated more of the processes into what I was doing, I found that essences were no longer needed. However, I have not "retired" flower essences from my work with this part of the nature kingdom. If they test positive as part of what a plant or entire variety needs for that last fine touch to balance, I'll be out there watering and spraying away.

There is one last thing. I have found, and so have many others, that if you pour any leftover solution that was made for you or anyone else in the family into the nearest potted plant, the plant seems to really like it. It grows, sometimes to silly proportions, and gets strong. It has nothing to do with whether or not this plant needs essences — it's just the reaction to flower essences in general. Or perhaps it's the brandy they like. At any rate, giving the leftovers to plants is an appreciated gesture. If you have a "sick" or weak plant and do not wish to plunge into the *Workbook*, try the random leftover solution-toss method. It might do the trick.

DEALING WITH ODD RESULTS

If you are using kinesiology or another related method for discerning which essences are needed, you will from time to time get results that look to be nuts. I do a lot of kinesiology testing, especially when working with flower essences. Most of the time — I'd say ninety-nine percent of the time — the results tend to fall within a certain range of patterning. But sometimes the results of a test look to be absurd. I'll do the testing, look at the results, look at the person, and think "This is crazy." I'll do the test again, making sure every aspect of the testing — my link with the person, my own essence balance, my focus, their focus, etc. — is clear. If I get the same results, I'll do whatever the testing indicates is to be done. I've learned that there are times when we simply do not understand on a conscious level what is going on. The kinesiology bypasses reason and logic, and links us in a way that allows the physical body to give us the input regarding what it needs, regardless of what we think.

I'll give you a very graphic example. I tested a woman who had had her jaw wired shut. She was having her jaw realigned. She tested for all twenty-six Perelandra essences — Garden and Rose — plus she was to put one drop of each concentrate into eight ounces of water and drink the entire eight ounces all at once. She was to do this every day for three and a half months.

I don't know if I'll ever come up with a more outrageous test result than this. I've never come even close. I tested myself to make sure I was clear. Then I tested her *two* more times, each time focusing with everything I had. During the second testing, I got a very clear, intuitive impression that people don't realize how extreme a jaw-wiring procedure is and the impact it has on the body and its balance. I also "saw" that wiring her jaw had restricted all movement along the spinal column.

I told the woman about the testing and my intuitive impressions. I also told her that the results were unusual. But I urged her, based on the fact that the results were obtained through kinesiology testing, to do this essence process.

For all of you who are asking, "Well, what happened?": She left Perelandra armed with the essences and saying that she would do the process for which she tested. I don't know the final outcome because I haven't heard from her. The points I wish to emphasize here are how odd the testing results can get and what to do when you come up with such results.

As for odd results during testing on myself: How do you think I developed all these different essence procedures?! I started out doing the basic flower essence test. That's it. The first time I did each procedure, I was moving forward on the basis of odd test results—which led me into entirely new ways to use the essences. I followed the test results, no matter how wacky, then saw the changes and felt their benefits.

And this is what I want to urge you to do. Verify your testing, of course. If the results verify, move forward and take the essences exactly as prescribed in the testing. This is how you will customize using flower essences to your personal needs.

It's also how we will continue to discover new and better ways of using the essences. I've been at this flower essence business for ten years now. As you can see, I've learned quite a lot. But I am convinced all the way down to my toes that we have only begun to scratch the surface when it comes to the potential uses and benefits flower essences have regarding health and life. (Partly, this is because we have only begun to scratch the surface on what "health" and "life" mean.) What I'm giving you in this book is a solid foundation, but this is not meant to be the final word on flower essences. Paying attention to your "odd results," following through with the essences, and observing the changes will add more information and keep us moving forward.

9

Hints on Buying Flower Essences

THERE ARE HUNDREDS AND HUNDREDS of flower essences available for purchase. You can buy a single bottle at a time or you can buy full sets of eight, eighteen, twenty-four, or thirty-eight. The bottles range in size from a dram (1/8 ounce), to a half-ounce, to an ounce. The way I have described the process for making essences is basically how all essences are made: a combination of flower petals, sun, water, and brandy. Then they are sometimes enhanced in various ways. I include mineral, genesa crystal, and tensor energies. I also include a direct partnership with the nature intelligences in the essence preparation process. For an idea of the current pricing range, refer to the order form in the back of this book.

What I'm trying to say is that there are a lot of essences available, all varying in size, quality, and production. And there will be even more available in the future. Every flower is probably a potential flower essence and no one person can make them all. If for no other reason, cost alone will require that a person approach the acquisition of flower essences with discernment.

My feelings, both as a flower essences user/practitioner and an essences producer, are that it is vital that each person have the essences they need available to them. I feel that flower essences should not be in competition with other flower essences and that each person must be able to obtain and use whatever sets or combination of sets they need in order to successfully enfold the essences into their lives.

I know that some who produce flower essences state that their essences should not be combined with essences produced by others. As far as the Perelandra essences are concerned, I do not agree with this policy and feel that you must be free to combine the Perelandra essences with whatever other essences for which you test positive. If a Perelandra essence combined with three other essences from three different "manufacturers" tests strong and positive for you, then I say combine them and take them.

In 1984, Universal Light gave me information that addresses this issue of discerning flower essences. Since I sometimes function as a flower essence practitioner, some of the information was addressed to this. If you are doing surrogate testing for family and friends, you are a "mini essence practitioner" and what is said applies to you also.

UNIVERSAL LIGHT

We will discuss the growing number of individual flower essences that are now being explored, developed, and even placed on the market. Everything that exists on a form level has healing properties or healing influence on at least one other thing on the form level. We are not saying that everything heals everything else; we are saying that everything has the potential to heal something. The grow-ing number of essences being discovered and made available is a result of, shall we say, not man's clarity but his confusion, his lack of groundedness. [Grounded: The full fusion of the soul within form (the body) and the resulting ability of the body/soul unit to function as one through form.] *When the soul is not fully stabi-lized within form, it becomes a more complex organism to relate to on a healing level; but as it becomes more stabilized, it becomes clearer—one can even use the word "simpler."*

There will be a tendency toward more (rather than fewer) essen-ces, but that will be temporary. What will eventually occur as man seats himself more fully into form will be the need for fewer essen-ces. He will find that where there were once twenty essences that ap-proximated a similar definition, that dealt with a similar kind of emotion with twenty different shades of differences, there will be one essence that will do the whole job. That is because his form in its more stable state will allow the one essence to be fully and com-pletely available to that form, and the essence will be able to deal with all twenty nuances of the emotion. Whereas you now have twenty essences dealing with twenty different shades of fear, you then will need only one which — containing within itself those twenty different aspects of fear — is fully accepted when it is introduced into the body. As man grounds, he will need less because he will accept more. It is a matter of quality rather than quantity. But for the time being, one will continue to see the phenomenon of many different essences put on the market.

A flower essence practitioner who deals with different kinds of people in varying states of groundedness will have no need to add indiscriminately to those flower essences that he already has. To accommodate people in different states of groundedness, we recommend that the practitioner discern those essences available to him that are the strongest within their own dynamic. For example, there may be twenty essences available that deal with the attitude and emotion of fear. Three or four within that group will sound a clearer note in respect to the dynamic of fear than the others, which will respond to areas of abstract subtleties. Those areas will be present in the three or four, but one might see them as secondary notes surrounding the principal note of each of those essences. Therefore, if a person needs help within the area of fear and is working with subtle dynamics, he will, in fact, respond to the note that also contains within itself the subtle dynamics. It is not necessary to break down fear into its twenty different areas and have every single note available to all people. However, because a practitioner deals with different levels of groundedness he will, in fact, rather than having one note, or essence, dealing with fear, need three or four. This is where his discernment will come in.

To add to this area of information, we would like to bring up the relationship of the essences to the practitioner — something not often considered. Remember, when healing, you are moving like within like on a horizontal level. There is a necessary relationship between the practitioner and the patient: Patients tend to gravitate to a practitioner of like mind. In order for the healing process to work most efficiently, one might say that the meshing of the practitioner and the patient must be "on."

In order to work efficiently, anything (any tool, device, product, or help) that the practitioner may bring to facilitate a healing process must respond to that meshing—not just to the patient, but also to himself. With the flower essences, the patient and practitioner are in a give-and-take situation. The practitioner's groundedness, his attitude, the development of his own emotions, and the condition of his own body all play into the communication process between him and the patient. In order for that process to work fully and efficiently, it is essential for the practitioner to draw to himself those essences that most clearly and fully are an expression of himself.

You will not have a practitioner with a collection of four hundred essences, even though it is quite possible for a practitioner to collect four, five, or even six hundred—the number of essences is going to expand enormously. But you will find practitioners who have different collections of essences. As this occurs, patients who are in need of essences will be drawn to those practitioners who most clearly resonate with their needs, their level of understanding and groundedness.

We are dealing with quality, rather than quantity. That to which the practitioner most clearly resonates can be translated into the essences, and the essence that most clearly and fully meshes with the practitioner will then be more clearly and fully available to the patient, as well. The clarity and quality of the essence, in terms of its effectiveness on the body, are related not only to the patient's level of acceptance but also to the practitioner's. Both of them affect the quality and effectiveness of the essence; both are confining and limiting or expanding and accepting the essences; and both affect the dimension and depth of the quality of that essence.

Okay. Let's get down to brass tacks here. You want to incorporate flower essences into your life, and you've just been told in a number of different ways that the essence world is your apple and before you lie hundreds, perhaps thousands, of essences from which to choose. There's a little "systems overload" if I ever saw it.

If you've been developing your ability to test flower essences as I've detailed in this book, you have the world's easiest solution to answering the question, "Which of these flower essences are for me?" Kinesiology! Here's what you do:

If You Do Not Now Own Any Essences

1. Get lists of flower essences from companies and societies that attract you favorably. Trust your intuition in this. I'm giving the addresses for the Bach Flower Essences and the Flower Essence Society Essences which, when combined with the Perelandra Rose and Garden Essences, will give you access to over 150 different flower essences. To get you started, I'll give you the list of the Perelandra essences.

Perelandra Rose Essences

Gruss an Aachen	Ambassador
Peace	Nymphenburg
Eclipse	White Lightnin'
Orange Ruffles	Royal Highness

Perelandra Garden Essences

Broccoli	Okra
Cauliflower	Salvia
Celery	Snap Pea
Chives	Summer Squash
Comfrey	Sweet Bell Pepper
Corn	Tomato
Cucumber	Yellow Yarrow
Dill	Zinnia
Nasturtium	Zucchini

2. Read through the list and the short definitions for each essence. Don't try to memorize the definitions. All you're doing is "feeding" the information to yourself, much like a computer. (You don't need to do this for the Perelandra essences since you've already read their definitions in Chapter 2.)

3. Ask:

Are there any flower essences in this list that I need to have available to me during the present period of time? (Test)

If you get a negative, go to the next list, read the definitions, and ask the same question.

When you get a positive, ask:

Should I have the full set on hand? (Test)

A positive response means you should have all the essences in that specific set on hand. They will be serving as your base. A negative result means only some are necessary, and you'll need to read through the list, testing each essence one at a time. You can ask each time or imply the question:

Do I need _____ essence? (Test)

As you go along, indicate or list each essence that gets a positive test result.

4. If you are going to be surrogate testing for family and close friends, look through the list again and consider other essences that may not be needed by you but would be by them. For example, if you have children, *you* may not need Snap Pea Essence (for nightmares), but your children might. For this, use common sense, intuition, and/or kinesiology. The question to ask (while you have in focus the people who you might test):

> Do additional essences need to be made available to this group? (Test)

If positive, or intuition and common sense are working clearly and you feel something is to be added, read through the list again, asking:

> Does _____ essence need to be added? (Test)

5. The results of all the testing will give you the combination of flower essences that will create your personalized set.

But don't throw the lists away. I suggest that about once a year (or more often if you intuitively feel the need), you check your set for possible updating. You will be changing and you may need additional essences in order to meet the new situations, challenges, and balance needs. The set you create now will be the base, the foundation, and this will remain operative for you throughout the road ahead. It's just that every once in a while you may need to add a couple bottles — or take away a couple.

If You Already Own Flower Essences

You'll be approaching your testing with the intent of updating and adding essences that are now needed in order to make your set current.

1. With the essences you presently own in front of you, ask:
   Are all of these essences still current for me? (Test)
A positive means these are still doing the job and remain as your base. If you got a negative, ask:
   Are *some* of these essences still current for me? (Test)
I doubt if you'll get a negative to this answer unless someone gave you a set of flower essences and you felt pressured to use them. In this case, that particular set may not be the one for you, and you'll need to consider other essences as your base.

If you got a positive, test each essence, one by one, asking:
   Is _____ essence still current?
With this test, you're just striking a note for efficiency and finding out which bottles you don't need to bother testing. Whichever ones are no longer current can be removed from the set for now.

2. Ask:
   Do I need to add other essences to my set in order to be current? (Test)
If you get a negative, you need go no further.
If you get a positive, go to your lists. Test each list separately. Read through the short definitions and then ask:
   Do I need any essences from this list? (Test)

Whatever lists test positive, read through all of the essences, one by one, asking:

Do I need _____ essence for my set? (Test)

The essences that test positive are the ones to be added.

Caution: Don't try to figure out the logic of the essences for which you test. They may be playing into patterns you don't realize are present—but you will! Within a year's time, I bet you'll be using the mystery essences and they won't be a mystery any longer. What you want to create is a full set of essences that is capable of addressing your current situation at a moment's notice.

I mentioned earlier that flower essences come in bottles varying in size—a dram to an ounce size, sometimes a two-ounce size. If you are planning to use the essences for just yourself and possibly a few friends or family, you'll need to purchase the small-size bottle. The larger sizes are for practitioners. At Perelandra we have only the half-ounce bottles in order to more efficiently accommodate everyone's needs. There are over 350 drops of concentrate in the half-ounce bottle—I actually counted, drop by drop—and since you use the concentrates one or two drops at a time, they'll last for many years. The concentrates are preserved in brandy, giving them an indefinite shelf life as long as you don't contaminate them. You'll know they are contaminated—this usually happens when a dirty dropper has been put back into the bottle—when little things are growing and swimming in the bottle. For those who are concerned about the brandy, we offer (special order) essences preserved in distilled white vinegar. They also have an indefinite shelf life.

To extend the life of your set even further, plan to mix solutions whenever specific essences are needed over an extended period of time. This way, instead of taking one drop of each essence concentrate every time, you can put a few drops into four ounces of water or make a solution bottle. Over a period of weeks you'll be using a total of perhaps five to nine drops per each essence concentrate in the solution rather than the twenty, thirty, or forty drops needed if taken as concentrates, a drop at a time, throughout the dosage period.

To make ordering from us easy, I am including in the back of this book ordering information for the Perelandra Essences.

10

Overlighting Deva
of Flower Essences
on Health and Balance

TO SAY THAT THE SURFACE *has only been scratched regarding flower essences and their role in the area of health is truly the proverbial understatement. If one is to look for the answer as to why flower essences work, one must be willing to look at the notions of health and balance first. And then one must be willing to turn upside down the presently accepted notions of health and balance and discover completely different concepts that address health and balance in new ways. Therein will lie the answers as to why flower essences work in such dramatic ways on the human body. And therein will lie the clues to the answers of many of the medical challenges for which, as of yet, you have no answers.*

"Health," according to the old notion, is the absense of illness. When nothing is wrong, when all systems are working, one has health. When illness or accident occur, one no longer has full health and addresses himself from the perspective of eliminating whatever is wrong.

"Health" in the newer light is the discovery and implementation of that which constitutes balance on all levels within a human system. Whereas the old focuses on the situation once health has been lost, the new focuses on the continuous process of what it is to establish and maintain balance within any given situation. In the old, when one is sick, he does whatever is necessary to eliminate the sickness itself. In the new, when one is sick, he concentrates on reestablishing balance, and as the body, mind, and soul restore that balance, the resulting adjustments eliminate any support on any level for the illness. In the old, the primary focus is eliminating illness. In the new, the primary focus is restoring balance.

We can look at the difference between these health concepts in another way. In the old, one has the tendency to look back, to look at his present state of health or illness in comparison to a past state of health. One's older years are compared with his younger years. In today's society health tends to be equated with youth. One is not as strong as he used to be. He is not as fit as in earlier years. He is not as lean as he used to be. He is not as lean as he **should** have been. He gets sick more often than he used to. People do things today for themselves in an effort to restore what used to be or what they think used to be.

In the newer concept of health, when one keeps his focus on balance, his concentration is in the present and his gaze is to the future. The concern is on what one must do to establish overall balance now and his willingness to modify his life practices in order to meet, adjust to, and strike balance in the future. Whereas the energy dynamic set up when one judges the present on the basis of the past renders the present stagnant or stuck, the dynamic set up when one focuses on the balance of the present with an eye to appropriate change in the future is evolution or forward motion.

*In the first chapter of this book, the principle of horizontal heal-
ing was discussed. At that time, the strength and effectiveness of
flower essences were explained as being due to the fact that healing
patterns concentrated within physical form (water and brandy) were
being used to balance and alter other physical form (the human
being). This is a universal principle, that the most effective sources
for health and balance within any given level or dimension can be
found within that very level. The fusion of the one to be balanced
with that which can impact in a balancing manner will be complete
when the principle of horizontal healing is adhered to.*

*Now, we take this principle a step further. (And in this present
age of quick change, this is only as it should be.) You are in a
period of transition. It is a universal phenomenon that presently includes all life and all reality on your planet and beyond. By definition, this requires change. In order to meet the challenges of this
transition, all structure, all systems, all form, and all fact must also
modify in order to incorporate the changes. This is the environment
in which you now live. Change and transition are the power and
force that presently surround you. To remain in tandem with one's
environment, one must internalize the surrounding dynamic of
change. This internalization is as it should be and gives you the support and strength needed in order to adjust yourself to the current
times. However much you resist the internal shifts required for you
to adjust and align to this time of transition will serve to separate
you from the principle of horizontal healing or, in other words,
horizontal compatibility. You will be an alien within your own
society and on your own planet. From you will resonate the vibration of that which used to be, while around you will resonate the
vibration of change. This will result in an inability on your part to
fully receive from the environment that which you need for health*

255

*and balance. You will experience friction and deterioration from
within and witness friction and the resulting deterioration of the life
around you. The principle of horizontal compatibility implies
synchronization and you will no longer be fully synchronized with
the surrounding environment.*

*But, let's assume that you have joined this time of transition and
that you are becoming synchronized with the intent and power surrounding you. The fact is, the vast majority of people on Planet
Earth have moved into the spirit of change. Each person will seek a
sense of comfort, security, and safety. One must have these things
in order to have the courage to change and move forward.
However, they will not be obtained by hanging onto the past, to
what one already knows. Hanging onto the past puts a person out
of step with this present dynamic of change and will only serve to
make him feel more uncomfortable, insecure, and unsafe. In this instance, the person has relinquished horizontal compatibility.*

*What will give one comfort, security, and safety, while all that is
around you is changing, is balance — internal and external balance.
The dynamic of balance is the key that you will hear repeated over
and over as people discover what is needed in order to move forward during this chaotic time. The foundation upon which comfort,
security, and safety will thrive will not be given to the individual
from sources outside himself, but rather will be created by the individual both from within and throughout his immediate surround-
ings.*

*You will see structures and organizations around you modify to
mounting pressures by reflecting a new attitude and intent on the
basis of balance. Facts that were considered bottom-line will be
reconsidered on the basis of balance, overturned, and will reveal a
new insight. From this, new reality will spring. Invention will*

flourish. Research will discover new vitality. All because the concept of balance was enfolded into and reflected through that which has existed.

On the surface, this issue of balance may appear to be a simple thing that should and could be initiated into one's life and environment in a relatively short period of time. If flower essences are barely understood, consider that the concept of balance is even less understood. If one needs an example, look to the problems of the natural environment for proof. Any concept such as balance, love, peace, reality . . . any such concept carries with it breadth and depth in ever-changing meaning and understanding. Balance will be a major key for the times we now face and for the lengthy period that lies ahead. Much is to be learned, explored, and changed in light of this concept, and souls will devote lifetimes on Earth to its exploration.

To return to the principle of horizontal healing or horizontal compatibility: You are getting the idea that all is changing. How one perceives his health is also changing. As with everything around him, the key to this change is balance. One's health will be intimately linked with one's understanding and response to balance. The body, mind, and soul are expanding at a rapid pace in order to remain synchronized with the surrounding overall universal dynamic of transition. There is a natural inclination within all life to respond to and within universal principles. If the larger picture is reflecting a new energy impulse, all life within that picture will automatically respond in kind, thus adjusting to and enfolding the new impulse. It is the natural seeking to remain horizontally compatible.

We come full circle. The reason why flower essences work so effectively within the human system is because of horizontal compatibility. The key to how they function is balance. They support and help secure balance on all levels — physical, emotional, mental, and spiritual. Physically, they balance the body by reconnecting and adjusting the electrical system. Emotionally and mentally, they help the person identify, alter, and sometimes remove emotional and mental patterns that challenge his overall balance. And spiritually, they assist the person's connection to and understanding of the many levels of himself so that he can operate in life from a broader perspective.

Flower essences provide a health system that is aligned to both the surrounding universal dynamics of transition, and the individual's expansion and response to the times by having incorporated within the system itself the key to it all — balance.

A Final Note about the Perelandra Flower Essences

The Perelandra Rose and Garden Essences are produced only by us here at Perelandra.

Also—and I don't know how to say this tactfully, so I'm not going to stumble all over myself trying—if you happen to see someone's shingle that claims this person is a recognized Perelandra flower essence practitioner, it's not true. We do not offer a practitioners' certification program; consequently there is no such "thing" as a recognized Perelandra flower essence practitioner. There is, however, a growing number of flower essence practitioners who are either self-taught or graduates from a sponsored practitioners' program, and who use Perelandra Rose and Garden Essences as part of their practice.

Bibliography and Resources

If you would like an international list of companies who produce flower essences, please send a self-addressed, stamped envelope to Perelandra.

Perelandra, Ltd.
P.O. Box 3603
Warrenton, VA 20188

W. Kapit and L. Elson. *The Anatomy Coloring Book.* 1993.
HarperCollins College Publishers
10 East 53rd St.
New York, NY 10022

DeCaro, Matthew. *The Gray's Anatomy Coloring Book.* 1980.
Running Press
38 South Nineteenth St.
Philadelphia, PA 19103

Flower Essences Order Form

___ *Co-Creative Science* $11

___ *Behaving as if the God in All Life Mattered* $12.95 **

___ *Dancing in the Shadows of the Moon* (hardcover) $23

___ *Perelandra Garden Workbook* (second edition) $19.95

___ *Perelandra Garden Workbook II* $16.95

___ *Flower Essences* $10.95 *

___ *MAP* (second edition) $14.95 **

___ *Perelandra Microbial Balancing Program Manual* $16

* *Flower Essences* is $8 when purchased with any set of Perelandra Essences.

** These books are also available in Spanish, see the Perelandra catalog.

___ Perelandra Paper # 4. Body/Soul Fusion Process $2

___ Free catalog of all Perelandra products

Perelandra Essences

___ **Basic Set**: Rose & Garden Essences (1/2-oz. bottles) $114

___ **Basic Dram Set**: Rose & Garden Essences (1/8-oz. bottles) $90

___ **Expanded Set**: Rose I, Garden & Rose II (1/2-oz. bottles) $152

___ **Expanded Dram Set**: Rose I, Garden & Rose II (1/8-oz. bottles) $115

___ **All Essences Set**: Rose I, Garden, Rose II, Nature
     Program & Soul Ray (1/2-oz. bottles) $228

___ **All Essences Dram Set**: Rose I, Garden, Rose II, Nature
     Program & Soul Ray (1/8-oz. bottles) $158

___ Perelandra Rose I Essences Set (1/2-oz. bottles only) $44

___ Perelandra Garden Essences Set (1/2-oz. bottles only) $86

___ Perelandra Rose Essences II Set (1/2-oz bottles only) $44

___ Perelandra Nature Program Essences (1/2-oz. bottles only) $50

___ Perelandra Soul Ray Essences (1/2-oz. bottles only) $44

___ Individual Rose, Garden & Rose II Essences $7.50 ea.
     (Available in 1/2-oz. bottles only. List below.)

_____

_____

☐ Please preserve my essences in vinegar instead of brandy.

Perelandra, Ltd. ✍ **P.O. Box 3603, Warrenton, VA 20188**
U.S./Canada: **1-800-960-8806** ✍ Overseas/Mexico: **1-540-937-2153**
Fax: **1-540-937-3360** ✍ Internet: **http://www.perelandra-ltd.com**

Send to (please print):

Name: _____

UPS Address: _____

_____

City/State: _____ Zip: _____

Daytime Phone: _____

U.S. Postage & Handling (International rates available on request.)

thru $8.00 . . . . $2.20	AK, HI, VI & PR:
$8.01 to 15.00. . . . . $4.50	Please send 1½ times
$15.01 to 50.00 . . . . $6.00	domestic postage. Your
$50.01 to 100.00 . . . . . . $7.00	package will be shipped
$100.01 to 200.00 . . . . . . $8.00	by first class U.S. mail.
$200.01 to 300.00 . . . . . . $9.00	
$300.01 and over . . . 3% of order	

Note: Prices and shipping charges subject to change without notice.

Subtotal: _____

Postage & Handling: _____

VA residents: + 4.5% sales tax: _____

Total: _____

Payment Method:
☐ Check ☐ Money Order ☐ Visa ☐ MasterCard ☐ Discover

Card Number: _____

Expiration Date: _____

Signature: _____

Credit card orders must be accompanied by signature.